CW01512682

American Medical and Sanitary Relief

in the

Russian Famine, 1921-1923

By Henry Beeuwkes, M.D.

Medical Director

American Relief Administration, Russian Unit

AMERICAN RELIEF ADMINISTRATION

Herbert Hoover, Chairman

42 Broadway, New York, N Y .

ACKNOWLEDGMENT

In the preparation of this report, the Medical Director wishes to gratefully acknowledge the assistance of Dr WALTER P DAVENPORT, Assistant Medical Director, who wrote several important sections, and of Dr JOHN E TOOLE and Dr HERSCHEL C WALKER for valuable assistance in its compilation

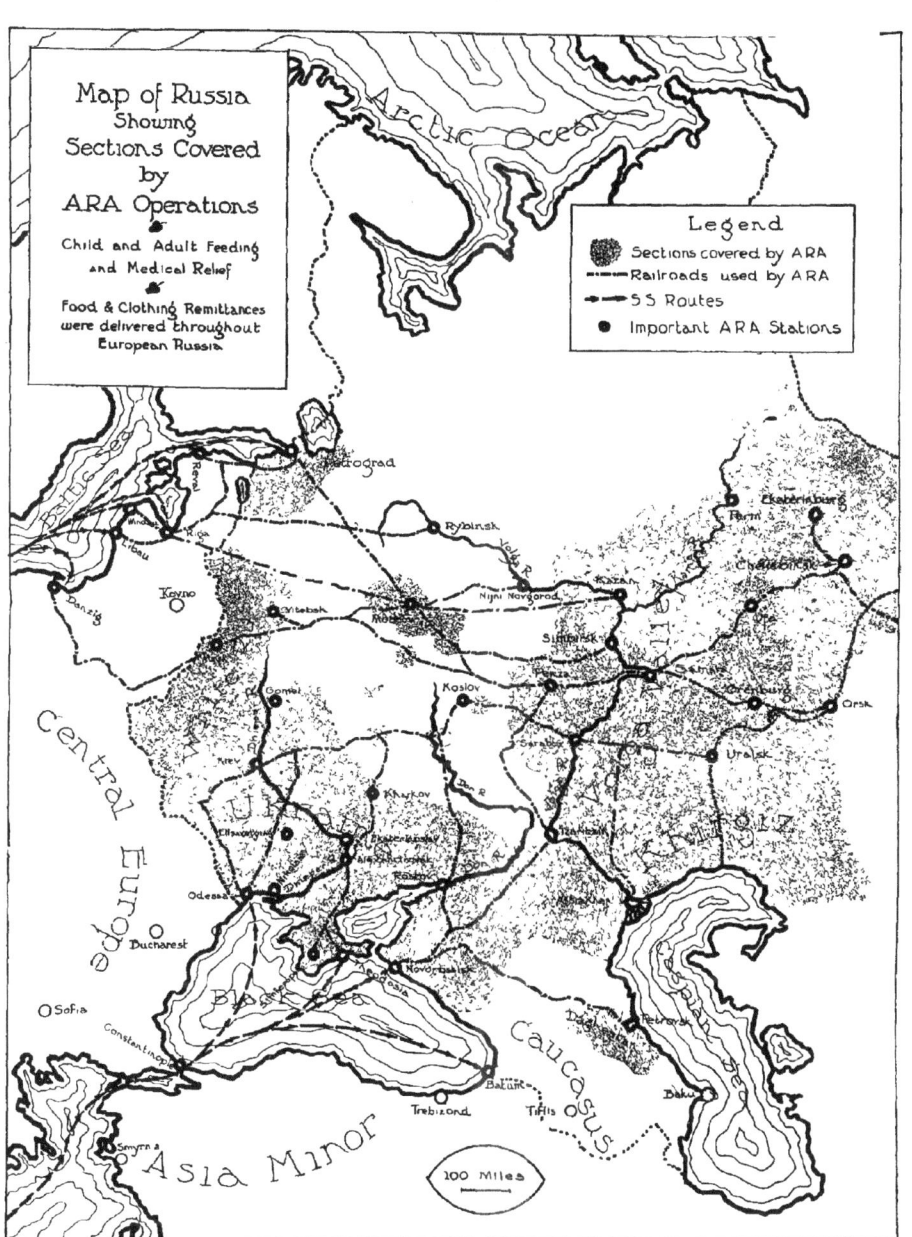

FOREWORD

Years of war, revolution and counter revolutions, prohibition of trade, paralysis of industries, disorganized transport, worthless currency, commercial isolation, destruction of homes, lowered resistance of the inhabitants incident to poverty, unhygienic existence and pestilence recurring with monotonous regularity, had so demoralized the Russian people that they were entirely helpless to cope with their new enemy which appeared in the spring of 1921, when complete failure of crops occurred throughout the Volga Basin and in the Southern Ukraine and threatened 24,000,000 persons with starvation and those scourges which always keep company with famine.

A signal of distress was sounded by the Soviet Government and it was promptly answered by Mr. Herbert Hoover, Chairman of the American Relief Administration. A "Russian Unit" was organized under the direction of Colonel William N. Haskell, United States Army, who had previously conducted relief operations for the American Relief Administration both in Transcaucasia and Roumania. The personnel of this organization consisted of members of the American Relief Administration, augmented by army officers and others experienced in relief operations. The first members of the Russian Unit of the A.R.A. arrived in Russia August 27, 1921. The visible resources at the time consisted of $9,000,000 for child feeding and $3,000,000 donated by the American Red Cross for medical relief.

Preliminary surveys of the so-called "Famine Area" by members of the Unit, made it evident at once that if wholesale death from starvation and disease were to be averted, greatly increased resources, both as regards food and medical supply, were imperative; that food reserves in the areas involved were practically nil, making necessary wholesale feeding of adults as well as children; and that the medical famine extended throughout Russia.

These facts were presented to the American people by Mr. Hoover and ex-Governor James P. Goodrich (of Indiana). Congress immediately donated $20,000,000 for food and seed grains and $4,000,000 worth of army surplus medical supplies. This gift, together with resources later made available by charitable organizations and individuals, finally provided a grand total of almost $60,000,000 for food relief and approximately $8,000,000 for medical relief. These gifts enabled America to rush food over seas and land to feed 11,000,000 starving Russian famine sufferers. The funds and supplies to combat the ravages of disease made it possible to give assistance to 5,764 hospitals with a bed capacity of 353,332, 4,123 ambulatories or dispensaries treating daily 247,087 sick, 4,760 children's homes harboring 336,821 children, 372 day nurseries with a capacity of 25,259, 165 schools and internats with 17,999 children, 248 homes for the aged and invalids caring for 59,237, and 987 other institutions making a total of 16,419 with a constant capacity of 1,039,735 persons. In addition millions of persons were inoculated against cholera, typhoid and para-typhoid fevers as well as vaccinated against small-pox.

This great American work started in September, 1921, and was brought to conclusion in July, 1923. Its magnitude and its unique problems of medical campaign and sanitation make the record of those phases, herewith presented, of interest not only to living readers, but to posterity.

This report has been issued in
two editions, the general edition
and a small special edition, the latter
being furnished only to qualified
members of the medical profession and
press. The special edition contains
representative photographs of disease and starvation manifestations.
Although thousands of such photographs were taken by members of the
American Relief Administration during
the famine, their abhorrent nature
is such as to make it seem desirable
to publish only representative examples.

TABLE OF CONTENTS
PART ONE

PART ONE

CHAPTER I

MEDICAL PRACTICE IN RUSSIA.

Medical practice was first encouraged in Russia during the reign of Boris Godunov (1598-1605). Foreign physicians were then freely permitted entrance into the country and a primitive Department of Pharmacy was founded. Before this time western physicians had been invited to Russia to serve as court physicians and also as diplomats. Mention is made in history of the beheading of a German doctor Bolarius, by Ivan the Terrible (1533-1584), because he was unsuccessful in effecting a cure in the case of one of Ivan's relatives. During the reign of the first Romanoff, Mikhail Feodorovitch (1613-1645), a Ministry of Medical Affairs was established and a drug store organized at Moscow, but medicines could be procured only by the Court and through personal petition to the Czar. His successor, however, permitted free sale of drugs and organized a second pharmacy.

Considerable progress was made during the reign of Peter the Great (1689-1725). This monarch took great interest in medical affairs, and officially invited Dutch and German physicians to settle in Russia for the purpose of teaching and practicing scientific medicine. During his reign he founded a "Surgical School" in Petrograd, which was transformed by Catherine into a Medical Collegium and finally became the Medical Military Academy. Peter also established the first free hospital for treatment of the poor in 1721, and in order to overcome the general distrust of physicians, he himself treated the sick and even performed minor surgical operations, wearing constantly at his side a small case of surgical instruments, and giving medical advice to all of his subjects. Peter also took many steps looking toward an improvement in sanitary conditions, replacing shops trafficking in poisonous medicinal weeds by authorized pharmacies. The Moscow University, the first higher institution of medical learning modelled upon European lines, was founded in 1755 and the Catherine Hospital was organized in Moscow during the same year.

Upon the accession to the throne of Catherine the Great (1762-1796) German culture in Russia received a great stimulus as she was a former Holstein-Gottorp princess. During her reign the Teutonic influence which predominated in court as well as in scientific circles, brought about a gradual advance in medical practice.

Not before 1861, however, when serfdom was abolished and the "Zemstvo" (1) came into existence, did medical assistance to the sick begin to emerge from its primitive state, and this is particularly true of the rural sections. Russian political administrative units consist of gubernias or provinces, correspond

―――――

1 The Zemstvo was in Imperial Russia an elected body of local rural government.

ing to our states; the cantons or ouyezds, similar to our counties; and the volosts, to our townships. There were small hospitals in the provincial capitals but the quality of medical work did not inspire confidence on the part of the population and charges were made for all medical attention, the only persons being treated gratuitously being convicts and soldiers. The serfs received medical attention only for very serious illnesses, and when discharged from hospitals were returned to their communities, a receipt being secured and charges for treatment demanded. Medical work in smaller towns and villages was under the supervision of local government doctors, but these were poorly trained, poorly paid, and so scarce that the peasant rarely saw them except upon the appearance of epidemics or when recruiting examinations were conducted. Medical work in the volosts was carried out by feldshers who on account of limited training were furnished with only a few simple remedies to treat the more common types of disease, most of their stocks of medicaments consisting of herbs grown in the surrounding country. Their work was controlled by a district doctor who made an inspection once yearly.

Such was the position of medical practice in agricultural communities when the work was undertaken by the Zemstvos, and all government institutions consisting of thirty-four provincial hospitals with 200 beds, and 303 ouyezd hospitals with 5,100 beds, were turned over to this organization.

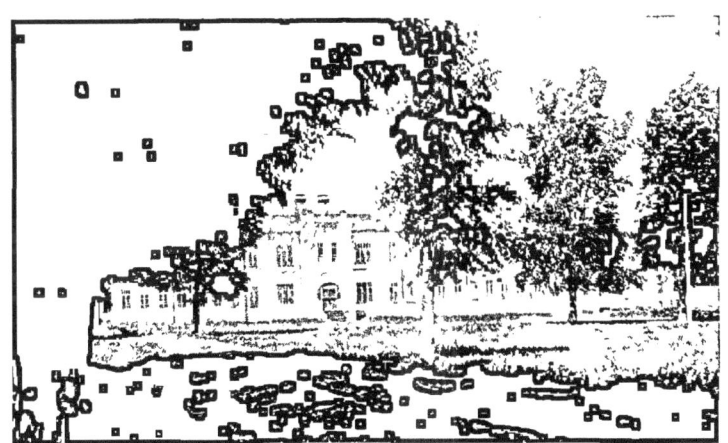

ONE OF THE BUILDINGS OF THE BLANDY MEMORIAL HOME, MIASS SIBIRIA
(In the Ufa District of the A R A)

This asylum re-established as a model children's institution, was re-named in honor of Harold Favielle Blandy, who died of typhus in this district while in the service of the A R A   Mr Blandy served from January until his death on May 17 1922

The Zemstvos or provincial Councils composed of representatives of the gentry, peasants, and town people were established in 1864, and all local health work, including the care of the sick was delegated to these newly formed administrative bodies. They had no judicial powers, but were concerned with all purely local administrative functions such as organization of schools, hospitals and dispensaries, construction and care of roads and bridges, and all measures concerned with the welfare of the population The funds required for the maintenance of the various projects were defrayed

-2-

by taxes which these bodies were empowered to levy.

Improvement in medical conditions could not be brought about at once after the end of serfdom, but only through a gradual evolution requiring many years The ignorance of the peasant had to be overcome as well as the prejudices of many members of the Zemstvo body itself, and education and persistence were necessary to overcome them. The Zemstvos began by degrees to improve and enlarge existing hospitals, and organize additional institutions in provincial cities and ouyezd towns

Improvement of the hospitals for the insane, a hitherto neglected phase of hospital work, was given special attention, and many such institutions were developed. By 1912, after fifty years of work, the Zemstvo had increased the number of hospital beds for insane patients from 1,167 to 26,000, wherein were employed 250 doctors especially trained in psychiatric work.

Previous to the time of the Zemstvos, very little attention was devoted to the sick village peasant, and this phase of relief work was now developed on an increasingly broader scale. In provincial hospitals a large number of schools for feldshers were organized and their trained graduates sent out into rural districts In every village of any size, or in the center of a group of smaller villages, a feldsher point, or ambulatorium, with two or three beds, was developed. These feldsher institutions fitted in admirably with the primitive living conditions existing among the peasant population. They were under charge of the feldsher or assistant doctor, who corresponds to a practicante found in our insular possessions

There are two types of feldsher, army and civilian; the army feldsher was usually selected from the annual incoming class of recruits, and after a two years theoretical and practical course of training in an army hospital, he could either serve in the army or go out into civilian life. The civilian feldsher, employed by the Zemstvo, was better qualified and trained, undergoing a three years course both theoretical and practical in the various feldsher schools operated in connection with Zemstvo hospitals. Before entering a feldsher school, applicants were required to have completed the first four years of the gymnasium course or its equivalent in the state schools. Despite the fact that custom and tradition placed the feldsher in a position superior to the nurse, and gave him a status of an assistant doctor, he was probably no better qualified to treat the sick than the average American male nurse He plays a very definite role in Russian medicine, and enjoys his distinct field because of scarcity of medical practitioners and the extremely scattered population

These Zemstvo feldshers were responsible for the medical care of all sick in their districts, and as their capability widened with training they were given an ever increasing armamentarium. Many of them became competent to handle even serious cases, either in the home of the peasant or at the feldsher point where a few beds were provided. Patients requiring surgical operations of any importance, and some of those suffering from serious disease were transferred to ouyezd or provincial hospitals. Zemstvo district doctors, one or other of the various ouyezd hospitals ᵉrvals, supervising and controlling the feld-ᵢions, they also treated the sick in consultation with the feldshers.

Though this was a very great improvement over what prevailed prior to the time when the Zemstvo took charge of the work, it never even approached an ideal. The number of district doctors was limited, and when they were mak-

-3-

ing trips of inspection, no one was left at the ouyezd hospital competent to treat the sick. At the same time, as the districts were very large, they were able to supervise and inspect the work of the feldshers only in a very general way, and were rarely available to give advice when difficult cases came up. Although many of the feldshers were poorly trained they were practically the only medical assistance available in rural sections.

There were, in 1913, 3,000 doctors in the service of the Zemstvos of Russia, 1,710 of whom had small hospitals in towns and villages throughout the agricultural centers. The total number of hospitals including ouyezd and provincial was 2,000 with a bed capacity of 45,000, and in addition, 26,000 beds were available for hospitalization of the insane. In addition villages of any size possessed a five or six bed ambulatorium. Local hospitals were almost always filled to capacity, each doctor treating from fifteen to twenty thousand patients yearly. As mentioned above, the more serious surgical cases were sent to the ouyezd hospitals, generally provided with infectious disease barracks, or to the large provincial capitals where excellent facilities were provided for major surgery and laboratory diagnosis. In many cases ouyezd hospitals were even more popular than the provincial institutions, due to the fact that doctors in charge developed considerable reputation along special surgical lines. In the town of Goli-Karamish, for example, with a population of 4,000, there was a fifty bed Zemstvo hospital which on account of the fame of the gynecologist in charge, drew patients from a radius of 1,000 versts, and in 1914 1,200 major operations were performed at this institution.

Before the World War Russia had a population of 140,000,000 people with 26,000 doctors, or one for every 5,400 of the population. These doctors were not distributed equitably, for in Moscow there was one doctor for every 1,000 people, in Kharkov one for every 700, whereas in Siberia there was only one physician for 60,000 people, and it was only through the agency of the excellent system evolved by the Zemstvo, that at least semi-professional care was made available for the rural peasant.

After the Russian revolution of 1917 the Zemstvos were abolished. Medical institutions were taken over by the new government, and placed in charge of the People's Commissariat of Public Health.

Prior to the revolution the Russian Red Cross contributed very largely to Russian medical relief. This organization was the beneficiary of special taxes levied on railroad and theatre tickets and the sale of playing cards, from which large sums were collected annually. Voluntary subscriptions were frequently large and members' dues added greatly to its income which in 1913 aggregated $130,000,000. The Red Cross organized, equipped and operated many excellent hospitals in provincial cities as well as in ouyezd towns, materially augmenting the work by the Zemstvo. At the same time large training schools were organized in connection with Red Cross hospitals and these furnished the largest percentage of practicing nurses During the World War this organization took a very prominent part in connection with hospitalization, treatment and after care of the Russian soldier. The Red Cross at present is under the control of the government, and although a certain amount of work was done during the 1921 famine and is still being done, through funds locally collected and contributions made by foreign organizations, it had lost its popular support and is no longer a very important factor in connection with medical work in Russia. The present Chief of the Russian Red Cross is also in charge of the medical work of the Russian Red Army.

MEDICAL EDUCATION.

Before the war, Russia possessed very good medical schools, located in Petrograd, Moscow, Kazan, Saratov, Odessa, Kiev, Uriev (Dorpat), Kharkov and Tomsk. The requirement for entrance to these schools was a diploma from a gymnasium given after eight years of study. There were two types of gymnasia in Russia: the "Real Gymnasium" which covered a seven years course in practical and technical work, emphasizing mathematics, science and the modern languages, preparing students for engineering and technical schools. The gymnasium proper required eight years study, provided a more classical course in which emphasis was placed on Latin and Greek, literature and, the modern languages and, in addition, elementary courses in physics, biology and botany. Graduates from the latter institutions were eligible for entrance to medical schools. Candidates entered medical schools, as a rule, at eighteen or nineteen years of age and after pursuing a course in medicine of five school years, of about nine months each, they were permitted to practice anywhere within the Russian empire. Most of the graduates accepted clinical appointments as externes in hospitals and clinics in the larger cities or provincial towns, and the Zemstvo and Red Cross hospitals selected medical personnel from among their number. Owing to the heavy mortality and great shortage of doctors incident to the World War, the medical course during that time was made continuous and shortened to four years.

After the Russian revolution and the establishment of the Soviet Republic, steps were taken looking toward the education of the working classes so that they might be able to take over the various administrative, technical and professional positions previously held by the bourgeoisie, and as a consequence educational institutions and measures looking towards the training of the working classes received a great stimulus. Workers universities were organized in practically every city in 1919, approved candidates being limited mainly to the working classes.

The "Rabotchy Facultet," workers university or "Rabfac" for short, in soviet parlance, was designed to take the place of the gymnasium. Such subjects as ancient and modern languages were eliminated to some extent, political courses emphasizing communistic principles being added in their place. The instruction given varies but is intensive and the students work hard during a course of three years. The special course, preparatory to entering medical schools includes geography, history, literature, mathematics, elementary physics and biology. The "Rabfac" is generally attached to, or affiliated with, a higher institution of learning, as a liberal arts, engineering or medical school, for which it prepares its students. When first established anyone from the proletarian classes, able to read and write, could enter the "Rabfac"; this is however not the case now, for a prospective candidate must now prove that he or she has been a worker for three years, and a member of the communist party. However, in some cases non-communists, provided they have proper recommendations from communists, or are able to pass a "Political examination" may be admitted. The political examination is especially designed to exclude anyone not desired.

Owing to the great need of physicians throughout Russia, the study of medicine was encouraged during the period 1918-1921, and communist medical students received rations and quarters. However, at the present time only fifty per cent of the students studying medicine receive government assistance and the great majority must augment their resources by securing some outside position while at the university. Candidates for medical school are now accepted on certificate from the "Rabfac," their preliminary training being assumed equivalent to that furnished by the pre-war gymnasium. Most of these young men and women enter on the study of medicine at sixteen and seventeen years of age; they are physically immature and for the most part possess very inferior preliminary training. While most of them are ambitious with great desire to learn, professors state that most students have not the capacity to absorb the material given them. This was officially recognized by a 1923 decree of the Peoples' Commissariat of Public Health requiring that elementary courses in chemistry, physics and biology be organized in all medical schools, indicating that the preliminary instruction in these branches was unsatisfactory. These students pursue a five years course of nine months each. Most of the graduates immediately go into practice in country districts because of the great shortage of doctors there.

It is believed that the present system of recruiting medical students has resulted in a distinctly inferior student body due to defective preliminary training. At the same time, medical schools, owing to lack of essential equipment, particularly laboratory supplies, microscopes, textbooks and literature, and the demoralized condition of teaching hospitals and clinics are not in position to give the most effective training. During the past six years, the teaching body has lost contact with developments in scientific medicine abroad, and as a result their teaching ability has deteriorated, while some excellent professors have been replaced by less competent communists. .

In 1918-1919 a special course was initiated to make feldshers eligible for practice, to fill the reduced ranks of physicians. The course was of three years duration and essentially practical and those enrolled received free rations, quarters and textbooks. But these courses did not produce very satisfactory results and were discontinued in 1922.

In spite of the great scarcity of qualified teachers and essential equipment to properly outfit teaching institutions after the revolution, medical schools were organized in many provincial capitals and there are now twenty-three in all of Russia, in which forty-two thousand students were studying medicine during 1922; 10,000 in Moscow, 7,000 in Petrograd, 5,000 in Kharkov, 4,000 in Kiev, 4,000 in Saratov and the remaining 12,000 scattered among seven provincial cities.

Russia finds herself at the present time[2] with a great shortage of doctors and with several thousand recent graduates only poorly trained. The situation is such that the Peoples' Commissariat of Public Health has announced, in a recent decree, that graduates will be required to attend courses at the various schools for special and more intensive work. The decree announces a shortage of 15,000 doctors and emphasizes the importance of training them during the next few years It states in addition that, due to scarcity of suitable teaching staffs, younger men, "politically" qualified and with suitable training, are to be nominated for the many vacant professorships which now exist.

Though great efforts are being made to increase medical personnel, and many continue to study for the profession, the lot of the doctor in Russia today remains a hard one. Physicians find it almost impossible to secure office space as many can scarcely house their families under the existing

----
[2] The present time throughout the report refers to 1923. Ed.

congested conditions. Medical apparatus lost, stolen or worn out during the war can not be replaced due to lack of funds, while relatively few persons have money to pay doctors fees so they apply for treatment at dispensaries. A large number of physicians have found it necessary to discontinue practice and take up more remunerative occupations.

THE PEOPLES' COMMISSARIAT OF PUBLIC HEALTH.

After the revolution and previous to the formation of the People's Commissariat of Public Health, the Zemstvo organization, which had been favorable to the revolution, continued to function, and other health agencies such as the institutions of the Russian Red Cross and the Union of Towns remained in operation. When the Soviet came into existence, they assumed charge of these institutions gradually eliminating many of the old officials who were replaced by communists. The Peoples' Commissariat of Public Health was established on July 21, 1918, as an integral part of the administrative machinery of the central government, under the Commissar for Public Health, who is a member of the Council of the Ministers of State and in a correspondingly forceful position to initiate and put into execution measures concerning public health.

All hospitals, ambulatories, dispensaries, sanatoriums, sanitary apparatus, laboratories, research institutions, pharmacies, dental dispensaries and children's homes, caring for children up to the age of three were nationalized, and placed under the administrative control of the People's Commissariat of Public Health, while the majority of the medical personnel including doctors, feldshers, nurses, pharmacists and hospital attendants were mobilized at the same time.

The new social Utopia was avowedly to afford its citizens medical care and everything necessary for their well being in both illness and health. In return, every citizen was to devote his services to the state. It should be remembered that for the great mass of the population, the principle of gratuitous medical treatment through the Zemstvos and similar organizations was well established, and as far as medical practice for the masses was concerned, this marked no great departure from what had been gone before. While private practice was not officially abolished, physicians suffered great hardships during this period, as those mobilized for employment in military, sanitary and civilian services, received little or no pay and the ration promised by the government was frequently not forthcoming, or only a small part of it received, sometimes several months after it was due. Those continuing in private practice were unable to gain a livelihood from the poverty-stricken population. Many physicians were forced to sell their furniture, pictures, medical libraries and eventually even their instruments, while others were forced to leave practice of medicine to take clerical positions in some government department.

After the creation of the Peoples' Commissariat of Public Health, but before the new regime was firmly established, political expediency played an important role in the policies of this department. It was only natural that men with communist party affiliations were selected to fill positions of administrative responsibility. Almost invariably they were absolutely unqualified and incompetent. Thus we saw feldshers and even veterinary feldshers in charge of provincial departments of health of large hospitals, and other medical units, directing the work of highly trained medical men under them with what detriment can be imagined. This also had far reaching effects in other fields: ambitious young doctors professing communism, in many cases secured preference over seniors whose political convictions were of another

-7-

color, and even in some cases succeeded them as professors, as chiefs of professional services, and on hospital staffs. Recently the authorities charged with these matters changed their attitude, and some of the better qualified medical men formerly in the provincial departments of health are resuming their old positions, nevertheless political considerations still remain an important factor in many appointments.

When the People's Commissariat of Public Health, or "Narcomzdrav", was first organized, a marked tendency showed itself for centralization of control of all public health activities throughout Russia, from Moscow through the provincial departments of health, i.e., the "Gubzdrav." The Gubzdrav, which functioned in the provinces, in turn had under their jurisdiction the ouyezd departments of health, or "Ouzdrav." Very little was left to the initiative of local health officials. Numerous decrees from the Center prescribed the methods to be followed in carrying out the work of the depart-

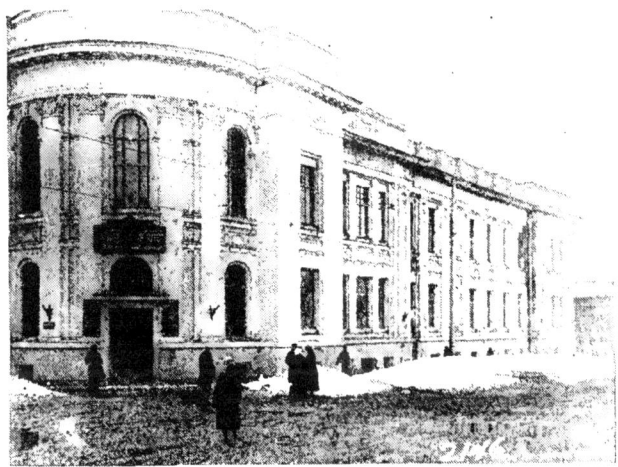

THE LENIN INSTITUTE, UFA, RUSSIA

ments as in hospitalization, selection and pay of personnel, combatting epidemic disease, and other public health measures. The methods of the Narcomzdrav were essentially bureaucratic and attempted to define work in exact and minute detail, more than often with no provision of the required funds, personnel or supplies. Child welfare work on a large scale was prescribed, but without providing sufficient milk; inoculation campaigns were ordered, but the materials furnished were insufficient; all cases of infectious disease were ordered hospitalized, but the number of cases far exceeded the bed capacity; delousing and disinfecting campaigns prescribed were impracticable because fuel, soap and disinfectants were not at hand.

When the New Economic Policy came into existence in the spring of 1921, the central government announced the withdrawal of all assistance to the local governments. Though this policy of decentralization was based on sound principles, the gubernias were left entirely without resources for the purchase of food, medical supplies or equipment, or even for the payment of personnel and fuel. As a result some hospitals and dispensaries were closed. Only continued assistance of the American Relief Administration prevented the wholesale elimination of medical institutions.

As most medical institutions are now operating for the greater part on local funds, administrative connection between Moscow and the provinces has been somewhat relaxed. Many hospitals and dispensaries were taken over by various factories, railroads, trading institutions and government syndicates, removing them from the control of the Narcomzdrav. The work of the People's Commissariat of Public Health became then largely advisory. However, efforts were made to tighten these bonds by appropriations from the central government to the provincial boards of health. Conferences are convened in Moscow, twice yearly, of representatives of health departments of provinces and autonomous republics. These provincial departments of health in turn convene ouyezd and district health conferences. A bulletin is also issued twice monthly by the Narcomzdrav, publishing official decrees concerning public health. The People's Commissariat of Public Health also publishes a monthly journal of hygiene and epidemiology.

The Narcomzdrav has greatly decreased its office personnel, but on the other hand, has increased the technical personnel; 5,500 persons now being employed in technical work in connection with public health as contrasted with 3,600 in 1917. In the field of epidemiology and bacteriology considerable progress has been made. An effective organization has been developed centrally and throughout the provinces, to combat preventive diseases, which should be a great factor in reducing disease, and controlling epidemics. The preparation of anti-smallpox, anti-typhoid and other vaccines are under state control through a special institute.

CHAPTER II
SANITATION IN RUSSIA
Sanitation in Russia has never reached that degree of development attained in Western European countries. The government itself took very little interest in the sanitary welfare of the population and no public health service, as such, existed. In the Department of the Interior at Petrograd a bureau of medical inspection for the collection of statistical data was maintained, which functioned through local representatives in the various provinces. The data on morbidity and mortality gathered for the "Crown" was notoriously unreliable and the methods in vogue were time consuming and bureaucratic. Chekhov in one of his stories, reports an outbreak of scarlet fever occurring in a school in the provinces. It was reported through various official channels to the statistical bureau in Petrograd, which issued a peremptory order closing the school. However, the order had to pass through prescribed channels, so that it reached the local authorities three months after the epidemic had subsided. According to prewar statistics four cents per person was annually spent for preventive measures against epidemic disease, and the total expended for all medical relief work was less than fifty cents per capita.

Sanitation in Cities.
Due to continued military operations and incident to the numerous civil wars, public utilities such as street railway systems, water supply, electric light and sewerage disposal plants, were temporarily thrown out of commission. However, they were functioning fairly effectively in some of the larger cities when the American Relief Administration entered Russia. Many of the smaller cities, even those possessing electric plants, remained in darkness and had recourse to small kerosene or sun flower oil lamps. Their water supply systems were not in operation due to leaking mains, broken down purification plants and lack of fuel to operate the pumps. Long lines of people waited their turns at water distribution points for hours, and even as late as August, 1922, water was sold by the bucket on the streets of Odessa. Other utilities were correspondingly demoralized.

The most adverse factors in connection with sanitation in cities, were the extreme congestion and the poor physical condition of buildings, plumbing and central heating plants, as well as the shortage of fuel and clothing. Many buildings have been destroyed; others of wooden construction have been wrecked to secure fuel; there has been no replacement by construction during recent years and repair work is only now beginning. In the city of Moscow there were in prewar times 27,872 homes containing 231,597 lodgings; at the present time there are 24,490 homes with 163,651 lodgings of which 60,921 are unsuitable for occupancy and all except 3,391 are in need of repairs. Of the 24,490 buildings mentioned above, only 9,682 are provided with running water, 6,500 are connected with the sewage system and 3,452 are equipped with central heating plants. The decreased housing facilities together with the influx of population into cities have taxed to the utmost all available accommodations, and families, formerly occupying a home or apartment, are now huddled together in one room.

Congestion in Moscow was even greater during the winter of 1922 than in 1921, for after a survey of apartments in the fall of 1922, the law permitting a maximum of sixteen square arshins(₁) per person was more strictly en-

---
₁ Arshin=27 inches.

forced and families were deprived of any rooms in excess of this allowance, additional persons being billeted in them. This maximum allowance was by no means enjoyed by the majority of persons. Frequently two or three persons live in a single room. I know of a family of six persons occupying one small room and others who live in corridors, closets, et cetera, which must serve at once as kitchen, living, dining and bed rooms. Congestion is increased during the winter as persons will frequently huddle together in the only room which they can afford to heat.

Family life has been more or less disrupted through these adverse living conditions, marked by worry, filth, congestion, poor food and a general lack of the ordinary comforts. The physique of the average individual has become depleted. This is manifested by anemia, lack of resistance and a marked increase in constitutional diseases, especially tuberculosis, which has grown extremely prevalent.

Fuel.

Until very recently wood was used exclusively for fuel. This was so extremely expensive as to preclude the operation of central heating plants where these existed Many individuals heated their rooms with a primus burner or small stove of brick and masonry. constructed in the center of the room, with a smoke pipe extending from a window or into the quarters of a neighbor, who accepted the smoke in order to secure the accompanying heat.

The hardships incident to fuel shortage can readily be appreciated when one realizes that Moscow, which is geographically at approximately the center of European Russia, has the latitude of Hudson Bay. In addition to individual discomfort and suffering, the lack of sufficient fuel, previous to the present year, was far reaching in its effects. Frequently it made necessary the closing of hospitals when infectious diseases were at the height of their incidence and when accommodations for care of the sick were taxed to the utmost. The effective operation of disinfecting apparatus was impossible for the same reason. Still more important was the scarcity of water caused by lack of sufficient fuel. In many cities water was available for only a few hours daily even for hospitals, and the bathing of patients was impossible. Owing to the lack of both water and fuel, bath houses could not be operated and the necessary laundry work was not done. People went for long periods without bathing or changing their clothing. This, together with a lack of soap, and the extreme housing congestion, made for a very high incidence of vermin infestation.

Though the supply of fuel remained inadequate and all our districts reported great difficulty in heating medical institutions because of fuel shortage, the situation was far better during the winter of 1922 than in the year before. Most individuals were able to secure enough wood to keep their living room considerably above the freezing point, and no longer found it necessary to sit about in overcoats and gloves as was the case the previous year. Also the number of hospitals which had to suspend operations for lack of heat was greatly reduced. Dr. Godfrey, the American in charge at Simbirsk reported that the peasants of Penza and other points, touched by our generous donations of medical supplies, brought loads of wood as gifts to the hospitals and homes.

Wood continues to be used almost exclusively for fuel, though some coal is used in heating larger buildings and considerable numbers of locomotives are now burning oil. Central heating plants of many buildings in larger cities have been repaired though the great majority of persons continue to heat rooms individually with small stoves.

-11-

Clothing.

Lack of appropriate and sufficient clothing caused untold suffering to a large percentage of the population. Comparatively little has been manufactured in Russia during recent years and imports have been extremely limited. Although the new economic policy permitted trading, stores and markets in cities have on hand considerable stocks of textiles and clothing, the prices of which are prohibitive for the average individual so the public must continue to make use of patched up prewar materials, or suffer for lack of them.

After the actual famine had subsided warm outer clothing appeared to be in even greater demand if possible, than food. The A.R.A. received constantly, from every district in which it operated, requests for underwear, shoes, stockings and outer clothing. Reports came in that many children could not visit kitchens, convalescent patients could not be discharged from hospitals, and children in homes were unable to take outdoor exercise because of lack of sufficient clothing. Any material which could be converted into outer clothing or undergarments was much sought after, including burlap bags and flour sacks.

Sanitation in Country Districts.

The peasant class makes up eighty per cent of the population. The peasants group themselves into small villages and conduct their farming operations from these centers. Most of this class are ignorant and illiterate and live the same primitive existence and practice the same primitive agriculture that their ancestors did in the 17th century. It should be remembered that only in 1861 was the peasant liberated from serfdom. The following story is illustrative: during the tercentenary of the Romanoffs, celebrated at Kostroma in 1913, the Grand Duke Nikolas Michailovitch, author of a number of serious historical works, said to the Tzar, indicating the thousands of peasants who stood before him: "These are exactly the same peasants as those of the 17th century who elected the Tzar Michael. They are absolutely the same. Do you not think that this is a bad thing?" The Tzar did not reply.

Sanitation in the smaller villages and country districts has not changed greatly within recent years, nor probably during the last hundred years. The peasant's home consists of a compound surrounded by a wooden, straw, thatched or mud wall and partly covered to afford protection for cattle. The buildings are limited, as a rule, to a barn for storage and a thatched cottage generally of one room which must serve for all the purposes of family life. Small windows light the room and there is no provision for ventilation. Furniture consists of a table and few stools, and occasionally a bed which is rarely used. A very large brick and mortar stove of domestic construction in the center of the room serves not only for purposes of cooking and heating but its broad upper surface, together with a platform constructed upon a level with the same, and just below the ceiling, provides a warm bed for the entire family.

Sanitary facilities in these primitive villages are non-existent. The water supply is derived from shallow open wells and the surrounding terrain is frequently badly polluted, no provision being made for the proper disposal of excreta. Piles of manure, refuse scattered about, and stagnant pools afford unlimited breeding places for flies and mosquitoes. Bed bugs and other vermin infest most of the homes. The primitive life of the peasant is in no way influenced by modern ideas of sanitation.

This comparatively low standard of sanitation which has always existed, and which was much aggravated in recent years has been responsible, in great part, for the high incidence of all disease and the terrifying magnitude of all epidemics.

HOSPITALS AND HOMES

The institutional facilities for the care and treatment of the sick were, previous to the revolution, reasonably adequate except in sparsely populated areas. They have already been described. Suffice to say here that many of the hospitals in the cities and even in the larger ouyezd towns compared favorably before the war with those in similar sized cities of Western Europe or America.

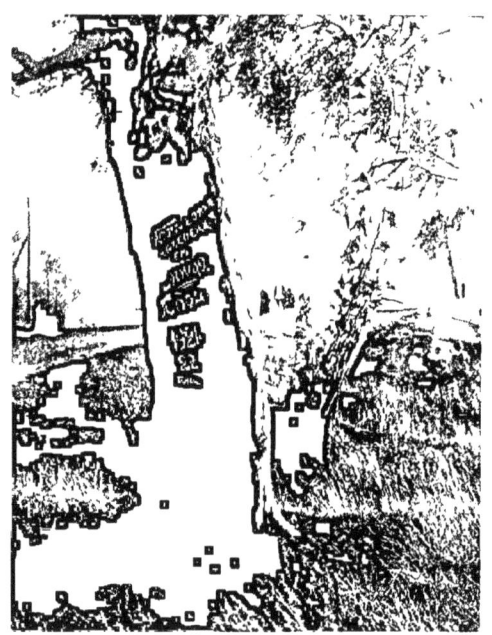

A LASTING SOUVENIR
The bark of this tree, where the inscription tells a lasting story, was eaten by the starving people of the Bashkir region in Russia. Bark formed a generally used food substitute during the famine

With the abolition of the Zemstvo by the revolution and the replacement of experienced medical administrators by inefficient political appointees, the efficiency of medical institutions dropped sharply. During the military operations incident to the various counter-revolutions, hospitals in the path of invading forces suffered very materially. Some were wrecked, and others more or less systematically looted of the various essentials needed by the military after the Revolution, little or nothing in the way of med- in Russia and imports gradually ceased. In to replenish expendable medical supplies or re- us that had become worn out, damaged or stolen. At the same time, funds were no longer available for the proper operation of institutions or to carry out necessary repairs, while the increasing exhaustion of resources caused by the famine of 1921 reduced all hospitals to much the same level.

As a consequence, inspections by Americans revealed hospitals in a most deplorable state. Buildings externally presented a dilapidated appearance, roofs leaking and plaster and woodwork falling to pieces. Wards and corridors were usually heated with improvised brick stoves as the scanty supply of fuel prevented the use of central heating plants, even where these had not been dismantled. The buildings were at times so cold that patients were frost-bitten and the drinking water at the bedside was frozen. The water supply and sewage disposal pipes were destroyed for the same reason, making it impossible to secure running water for the use of the toilets, lavatories and bath-rooms.

The wards could not be properly ventilated due to the shortage of fuel and a heavily foetid odor characterized hospitals everywhere. Beds were fairly substantial but a large proportion of the mattresses were worn out. Sheets and bed linen were generally absent, while the only clothing for patients often consisted of their own underwear. Blankets averaged one per bed but many of them were worn out or of such poor quality as to be practically worthless. Bedside equipment consisted of little beyond a broken glass or tumbler or a rusty tin can. Other ward equipment, such as bed-pans, urinals, and especially rubber goods and thermometers, was either absent or inadequate. Mess equipment was as scarce as was food for patients. Many of the patients, therefore, upon entering the hospitals, brought with them their own mess utensils, bed linen and frequently their own food.

Surgical pavilions were in particularly bad shape. Sterilizing apparatus had to be improvised to replace the large steam sterilizers that were either broken down or not to be operated because of shortage of fuel. Chloroform and ether were so scarce that at times it was necessary to perform operations without anaesthesia. Among the army surplus medical supplies, the A.R.A. received a large quantity of chloroform, a small proportion of which had deteriorated due to long storage and we accordingly issued it--"For External Use Only " In spite of this fact, it was used in several districts for anaesthesia and pronounced superior to any furnished by the government. There was a great shortage of surgical dressings, and gauze, while bandages were seldom seen. In many hospitals operations could be performed only on condition that the necessary dressing material be supplied by the patients. Surgical dressings were used over and over again and large superating wounds and faecal fistulae were frequently dressed with old newspapers or any other material that could be procured. The supply division of the Health Department of Samara received 220 yards of surgical gauze during the year of 1921, to meet the needs of all medical institutions throughout the province which numbers 3,000,000 people. There was a great lack of suture material as well, and one of the leading surgeons in Simbirsk informed us that he frequently used thread, drawn from old clothing, for the closure of surgical wounds.

Inspections of the drug and stock rooms revealed mainly empty containers; essentials such as quinine, aspirin, neo-salvarsan, bismuth, the bromides and digitalis were almost universally absent and the few stocks remaining on hand, even in larger hospitals, could generally be stored on one or two shelves of a small cupboard

The great shortage of fuel, soap and other disinfectants, and even of water, made it impossible to bathe patients on admission in many hospitals or even to disinfect the clothing of those suffering from infectious diseases. Their receiving pavilions were alive with vermin and lice with which patients were infested.

The food for patients supplied by the government was inadequate and inappropriate for feeding the sick. Preparation of suitable diets was out of the question, the only aim being to secure nourishment enough to keep patients alive. Food for personnel generally consisted of one pound of black bread per day.

Some of the institutions in larger centers were in a much better condition, both as regards equipment and supplies, and carried out reasonably effective work without our assistance. These were however, decidedly the exception and the need for essential medicines as well as for bedding, blankets, soap and disinfectants was universal.

The personnel in most of the hospitals was decidedly greater than that required to take care of patients the attendants frequently equalling the number of sick in the institutions of the famine area. These attendants as a rule received no pay beyond the very scant ration of black bread, but as this was their sole opportunity to avoid starvation, they were only too willing to work without other remuneration. The surplus personnel made for diminished administrative efficiency and at the same time they had a tendency to augment their ration by appropriating some of the meagre food provided for patients. Doctors, nurses and attendants working under filthy and demoralized conditions, with scanty supplies for treating the sick, many of them on the verge of starvation, had lost their enthusiasm. Practically all medical personnel had contracted one or several of the various infectious diseases surrounding them on every hand, and great numbers had died. The morale of the survivors was at the lowest ebb.

Hospitals at this time presented most deplorable pictures. The filthy sick who applied in overwhelming numbers and could not be bathed or supplied with clothing, were frequently seen two or three in a bed. At times the dead lay among the living. Under these conditions many patients preferred to die at home without medical attention. Nevertheless the numbers admitted to hospitals were frequently double the capacity of institutions available to receive them.

Dispensaries.

Few dispensaries, likewise, had medicines to issue, physicians simply examining patients and issuing prescriptions. In local pharmacies stocks were meagre and prices so high that the majority of persons were unable to get their prescriptions filled. This necessitated the opening of dispensaries and pharmacies by the A.R.A., where prescriptions were filled gratuitously for all poor.

Some of these dispensaries were poverty stricken beyond words and at one of them visited by Dr. Ross a large sign was posted stating that all those requiring medicines must bring their own paper for prescriptions. Almost invariably those needing surgical operations were required to supply their own dressing material.

Laboratories.

Laboratories suffered as well from the general supplies shortage. Large quantities of cholera and typhoid vaccine were being prepared, but the production of biological products requiring animal immunization, such as diphtheria anti-toxin, smallpox vaccine and various sera, had fallen to almost nothing. When we visited the Roux laboratory in the fall of 1921 we found them bottling some diphtheria anti-toxin which had been prepared two years before, but no other work was being done. The laboratory was actually not operating because culture media and other laboratory supplies were not available. No animals were at hand for inoculation, nor was water, fuel or food for personnel. Their many wants were soon provided for and they have for a long time been manufacturing large quantities of biological products.

The effectiveness with which large laboratories were operating in Russia depended of course on the ingenuity and initiative of those in charge of the work. While the laboratory at Samara produced nothing, that serving the Ufa gubernia was manufacturing considerable amounts even of smallpox vaccine, although the economic situation in Ufa was in no way more favorable than that existing in Samara. Most of the laboratories had been organized on a pretentious scale, provided with every variety of expensive apparatus, but expendable articles such as material for making culture media, stains and all varieties of glassware were everywhere in great shortage.

Children's Homes.

Under orthodox communistic principles, men and women, fathers and mothers alike, were included in the category of workers, and the children were to be cared for, reared and trained by the state in children's homes and other institutions. Though this principle was not carried out in practice, the Soviet Government has shown an extraordinary interest in child welfare. The Government requisitioned and converted into children's homes many of the finest buildings in all cities. These are of two sorts, one for infants below three years of age under the jurisdiction of the Narcomzdrav, and the other for older children in charge of the Department of Education. There are also great numbers of nurseries where children are cared for during the day while their mothers are at work.

Great numbers of children have been thrown upon the mercy of the government during recent years; many of them were left orphans by war, revolution, and epidemic disease. Others were lost during the refugee movements, or deserted by parents no longer able to care for them.

The problem of handling thousands of deserted, lost, and orphan children throughout all famine areas was very difficult. Local resources were utterly unequal to the needs. Homes were established where all children picked up upon the streets and roads or in railroad stations were housed for a certain number of days, after which they were forwarded to permanent local homes or shipped in carload groups to other points. These receiving homes were little more than death traps. Hastily developed as the increasing number of waifs demanded, they were without sanitary facilities. Their condition was beyond description. Five such receiving homes were set up in Samara city and a corresponding number in other towns, each housing thousands of children. The capacity of these institutions simply equaled the numbers who could be huddled together upon the floors. The buildings were without furniture, the rooms were unheated, and there was no underwear or outer clothing available to replace or augment that which the children wore when admitted. There was little provision for bathing and no facilities for delousing or disinfecting their vermin infested clothing. There were no toilet facilities, and the grounds about the buildings and even the floors of corridors, hallways and rooms were strewn with dejecta. Here in these homes one saw the most advanced horrors of starvation; children in most extreme stages of anemia, others living skeletons and many swollen and puffed with edema. An attempt was made to segregate those actually ill, but under the congestion existing, and with lack of medical facilities, segregation could not be effectively carried out. Thus many children contracted infectious diseases or died of starvation before they could be disposed of. These receiving homes were gradually eliminated or reorganized with the help of the A.R.A. and replaced in many cases by model institutions.

The "Detsky Dom's" or permanent homes, even in the famine areas, were
in far better condition than the makeshift institutions receiving homes. But
as the number of waifs was tremendous and facilities very limited, they were
overcrowded, and many of the children remained infested with lice due to lack
of cleansing and delousing facilities. Little or no clothing could be provided and many children were naked. One frequently saw three or four little
children under a single worn-out blanket. Many buildings were not heated and
sanitary appliances were generally lacking. With the assistance of the A.R.A.
the supply of bedding, blankets, soap and other disinfectants, cod liver oil,
medicines and bedside equipment, and most important of all, a supplemental ration, they became able to care for the children in a reasonably satisfactory way. Some of them even became model institutions.

The organization for the care of children leaves much to be desired,
as present methods are wasteful both as regards personnel and housing facilities. In Moscow and other large cities where congestion is general, many
large buildings are set aside as children's homes and harbor a few children,
the personnel frequently equalling the number of inmates. Day nurseries which
care for forty children for eight hours a day, frequently support sixteen
adult attendants, while in one home in Moscow with one hundred children the
staff consists of ninety adults. Some economy in this respect is being
brought by the consolidation of numerous small homes. This reduces overhead
expenses, which must facilitate training and education in larger units.

CHAPTER III.
FOOD CONDITIONS.

Previous to the spring of 1921 the government prohibited all trading and compelled people to exist on a "paiok" (or ration) which it tried to supply, and which could only be augmented by secret trading. Only those registered as "workers" were eligible for a ration.

As there were no private enterprises, all workers were government employees. This class included, among many others, government officials, those employed in factories, laborers, school teachers, physicians working in hospitals, and the multitude of clerks employed in the government offices.

All workers received in the beginning an equal paiok, irrespective of the position held, or the quality or quantity of work performed, the only requirement being registration. Many of the bourgeoisie, who were not carried as workers or students, had to perform manual labor such as shovelling the snow, or cleaning the streets at irregular intervals, for which they received a pound of black bread daily. At a later period departments began to vary the paioks, some furnishing a much larger ration than others. Those issuing the best ration were naturally the most popular. Many performed little service, while others registered in several departments and secured double or triple paioks. Government employees were finally classified into categories according to the character of the work which they performed. Highly skilled workmen and government officials received the largest paiok regularly, while the size of the ration supplied those in the lower categories varied with the amount of food available and was less regular in its issue.

The academic paiok went to doctors occupying positions of responsibility, professors, and scientific men, and those eligible for this ration were given, in addition, one-half ration for each member of their families unable to work. Other categories included hospital patients, invalids and soviet employees. The distribution to them was irregular and the size of the issue smaller. Those not registered received only an occasional issue of flour or potatoes. Children, students and nursing mothers received special consideration. As a matter of fact, the paiok which the average individual received was insufficient in amount and entirely unsatisfactory from the point of view of quality and variety, and so uncertain in its issue that during the winter of 1919-1920 a large proportion of the population were subsisting on little besides frozen potatoes, black bread and occasionally a little cabbage or fish. Secret trading went on in spite of the prohibition. Some food could be purchased from cooperatives and even a limited amount in the markets and near railroad stations, where "bagmen" congregated and traded more or less under cover. Thousands went into the country to barter household goods, jewels, furs and clothing for a little food.

The prohibition of trade made it impossible for the peasant to dispose of his products to advantage, and the policy of the government of taking the crops and giving him nothing in return discouraged farming operations. The farmer therefore reduced his acreage, planting only a sufficient amount for the needs of his immediate family. The crop total accordingly fell and when the famine developed in the fall of 1921, involving the entire Volga and Southern Ukraine areas, only meagre surplus stocks of food existed in this area or in other parts to make good the shortage. The sections involved in famine were the great grain producing areas of Russia. Reserves of grain, sufficient for one year, which the farmer attempted to keep on hand to safeguard against famine, had previously been requisitioned for the armies or consumed.

The population of the famine area as estimated by the Soviet Government in the spring of 1922, together with adult and child population classified as "Starving" is as follows:

	Total Population.	Starving.	Adults.	Children.
Volga Provinces...........	32,691,000	20,215,000	11,109,000	9,106,000
Ukraine (famine sections).	9,655,000	3,680,000	1,786,000	1,894,000

It is difficult to give an estimate of the numbers who would have died, had it not been for the generosity of the American people, who through the agency of the American Relief Administration furnished food to a maximum of over 10,000,000 people daily Undoubtedly millions would have succumbed. It was very difficult to differentiate between deaths from famine and disease at a time when epidemics were carrying off great numbers of the population and large proportions of them were without adequate medical attention

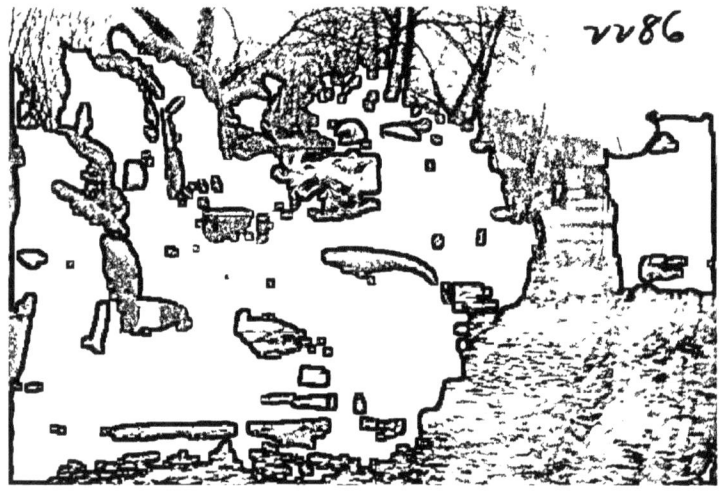

COLLECTION OF FAMINE VICTIMS
Corpses gathered in by Red Soldiers from wherever victims happened to be at their last moments

Under the "New Economic Policy" of 1921, permitting trading, considerable stocks of food and clothing appeared in the markets and in stores opened either by private individuals or by co-operatives, so that even in cities throughout the famine area a fair quantity could be purchased. However, prices of food rose out of all proportion to the salaries of a great proportion of individuals, and most persons remained chiefly dependent upon the ????? which the government continued to issue.

????? at 68,000 rubles to the dollar upon the ar-
1921, and by November of the same year it had
????? cially, as much as 300,000 rubles per dollar
were being paid. The average salary at the time, even in Moscow, was only 600,000 rubles per month, while flour cost 16,000 rubles, meat 18,000, sugar 50,000, butter 50,000 to 60,000 per pound and milk cost 10,000 rubles

-19-

per pint. It is quite obvious that food shortage and misery existed far beyond the actual starvation areas and involved gradually even those who were fortunate enough to live in the metropolis. People in cities and towns increased their resources by selling anything that they could dispose of. The streets about markets were crowded with people offering for sale their household effects, overcoats, bonnets, toys, jewels, ornaments, furs and what-not. However, acute starvation was limited to the provinces and especially to their rural sections.

Famine Areas.

Large numbers of persons in the famine areas sold their belongings in order to augment their food supplies and slaughtered their cattle in order to procure food, or because they were unable to feed them. Many others forsook the unfortunate sections and began mass refugee movements. As the meagre food supplies vanished, they had recourse to all kinds of food substitutes.

Food Substitutes.

Incident to the numerous famines that have occurred in Russia, the people have learned to use many substitutes which, though not actually suitable for food, may take the place of it when the latter is not obtainable. These are of two general varieties: one class made up of substances with a certain amount of food principles, the other entirely devoid of the same and used only to avoid the discomfort which accompanies an absolutely empty stomach. "Lebeda," a weed which grows more or less universally throughout Russia in gardens and rye fields especially when the crops are bad, is the most commonly used substance of the first class. Its chemical analysis shows approximately ten per cent of water and ninety per cent of dry substances, the latter consisting of seventeen per cent of nitrogeneous matter, seven per cent of fats, forty-nine per cent of starch and other extractives, and twenty-one per cent of soluble tissues and five per cent of ash, but it is more or less indigestible and unadaptable for food.

Those feeding on this substitute soon become exhausted and develop symptoms indicating that the weed has toxic properties. As the crop of lebeda was scanty and quite expensive, it was frequently adulterated with acorn flour, bark of trees, rushes, hazel-nut tufts, the husks of seeds, potato-peel, sawdust, wild rose, the leaves of a great variety of trees as well as grass from the fields. Finally, when those substitutes were exhausted, the peasants collected bones and ground them up into flour. First these substitutes were used to adulterate meagre stocks of rye or wheat flour. In the end when these were exhausted, bread was made exclusively of adulterants. A white clay resembling stone, containing a small proportion of organic matter, was also extensively used as an adulterant for making bread throughout the Volga area. In numerous villages which I visited during the spring of 1922 many families made bread exclusively of bones, rushes and clay. This "bread" was the only food remaining on hand up to the arrival of American corn.

Cannibalism.

Dogs, cats, rats, and other rodents were eaten by the starving people, late in 1921 rumors of cannibalism began to reach us. Many authentic cases of parents killing and devouring their children were soon definitely established. Murders were also committed and the bodies of the victims used for food. Conditions grew worse, and the practice of eating those who had died of disease or famine became constantly more and more frequent.

In connection with cannibalism, the investigations of Professor Frank of the Department of Mental and Nervous Diseases, Kharkov University, concerning the mental abnormities of reported cases of cannibalism are of interest. He investigated all rumored cases in the gubernias of Odessa, Donetz, Zaporozh, Nicolaev, and Ekaterinoslav and established the authenticity of twenty-six cases in which human beings were killed and eaten by their murderers. He also found seven cases in which murder was committed and the body sold for pecuniary gain, the flesh being disguised in the form of sausage and placed upon the open market. He found the practice of necrophagia very common. At the time I visited Orenburg a law had just been passed permitting the sale of meat only in bulk form, so that it could be identified, in view of the fact that considerable amounts of human flesh had been sold on the markets. Probably a great proportion of the cases of cannibalism were incident to abnormal mental conditions on the part of the starving population, for in addition to the typical "Deficiency Diseases," which will be discussed later, the various manifestations resulting from famine conditions may be classified as follows:

1. Simple cachexia--gradual exhaustive loss of weight and strength, loss of appetite, dullness and apathy. Individuals lose hope and often, in this state, desert their homes and children, and go they know not where "to await death to come in accordance with the will of God." Some develop maniacal symptoms, becoming like wild animals and at times practice cannibalism.

2. Cachexias associated with dropsy and albumuria.

3. Cachexia accompanied by great gastro-intestinal irritation, diarrhoea, and frequently polyneuritis. The diarrhoea may be so severe as to resemble cholera. There is the suggestion that this may be due to some special intestinal bacterial flora existing in this type of cachexia, which is very malignant.

The lack of food and the use of food substitutes began to show their effects early in the fall of 1921, and conditions became rapidly worse during the winter and early spring and up to the time of the arrival of the American corn. Starving persons drifted into cities and towns, gathered in refugee camps, collecting homes and hospitals, where they continued to starve on the very meagre rations supplied by the government. Over 7,000 waifs were collected in the streets of Kazan alone during the month of November, while 22,000 were at this time being harbored in homes of the province of Ufa. The incidence of disease was naturally extremely high and the mortality rates of some of these institutions reached thirty and even fifty per cent for a single month. Many died on the roads en route from country districts to cities, and dogs, birds and other animals devoured their bodies. A large number died after arrival, upon the streets.

Decent burial of the dead was entirely unpracticable and I saw as many as 500 bodies collected in the morgue of a single large general hospital; great pits were being dug and all city dead, gradually collected, were piled naked in tiers within these pits until they reached almost the ground level, when they were covered with a superficial layer of earth.

The medical situation was extremely difficult at this time, the famine conditions producing a tremendous amount of sickness and at the same time preventing proper care of the sick. Medical personnel were practically starving, hospitals were without supplies, without fuel, and most important of all, without food. The government ration for patients was theoretically meagre enough, the allowance in Kazan being as follows:

```
Black bread.. . . . . . .1 pound    Cereals.......... ...... ¼ ounce
Meat.......... . ...    .2 ounces   Sugar.. ................24 grams
Fat...... . ........ .  1 ounce
```
The paiok of the personnel consisted of:
```
Black bread............1 pound a day
```
        This ration was, however, merely theoretical and the actual amount
of food received by hospitals fell far below the figures quoted, so that in
many hospitals patients received only a thin soup and a little bread daily.
In the Samara gubernia, the government supplied only 2,000 rations for 11,000
beds. The shortage of foods, fuel and supplies, the constantly threatened
closure of a large proportion of institutions. The American Relief Administration allocated thousands of supplementary rations for sick in hospitals,
as well as for the general child population. After the arrival of the American
corn the A.R.A. supplied institutions with all their medical and surgical
needs, their patients with food, their personnel with corn, and their physicians
with the food and clothing packets, donated by Mr. William Bingham and others.

GENERAL FOOD SITUATION

        The following regions were registered by the government as famishing
in the winter of 1922:

Votsk Oblast
  Glazov Canton
  Debess Canton
Tartar Republic
  Spassk Canton
  Sviajak Canton
  Bouinsk Canton
  Tetiushi Canton
  Chelny Canton
  Chistopol Canton
Tchuvash Oblast
  Tzivilsk ouyezd
  Cheboksari ouyezd
  Batirevzk ouyezd
Penza Gubernia
  Gorodishe ouyezd
Samara Gubernia
  Melekes ouyezd
  Pugatcheff ouyezd
German Communes
  Markstadt ouyezd
  Krasnoyarsk ouyezd
  Tolkeshurovsk ouyezd
  Krasni-Kut ouyezd
  Poltava ouyezd
  Polotzk ouyezd
  Rovnoy ouyezd
Saratov Gubernia
  Dergatchevsk ouyezd
Tzaritzin Gubernia
  Lenin ouyezd
  Nikolaev ouyezd
Kalmuk Oblast, wholly,

Bashkir Republic
  Usergunovsk Canton
  Burzian-Tangourovsk Canton
  Kip-Djetirsk Canton
  Urmatinsk Canton
  Argayshaky Canton
  Tamian-Kataisk Canon
Tcheliabinsk Gubernia
  Verhne-Uralsk ouyezd
  Miassk ouyezd
  Tcheliabinsk ouyezd
Morgolsk Oblast
  Selegunsky Aymak
Fergana Oblast, wholly,
Daghestan
  Andisk region
  Avarsk region
  Gunibsk region
  Samursk region
  Kazikumuksk region
  German Commune of the region of
  Khasaturoff
Armenia, wholly,
Crimea, wholly.
Ukraine
  Melitopol ouyezd, Zaporozh gubernia
  B. Tokmak ouyezd, Zaporozh gubernia
  Dnieper ouyezd, Nikolaev gubernia
  Odessa ouyezd, Odessa gubernia
  Kargopol ouyezd
Vitebsk Gubernia
  Velikye ouyezd
  Lepelsk ouyezd

Kirghiz Republic   Gorodoksk ouyezd
  Boukeevo gubernia   Polotzk ouyezd
  Uralsk gubernia

This does not mean that widespread starvation existed in any of these
areas, but rather that the food available was below the nominal needs of the
population. In some of them great shortage existed, and as the available resources became exhausted there was considerable suffering and some actual
starvation, especially in inaccessible and isolated areas where seed grain for
spring ploughing arrived too late, or in insufficient amounts, or where shortage of animals had made the tilling of sufficient acreage impossible.

In other sections food remained fairly plentiful throughout the winter and the markets of cities were well stocked with staples. The prices of
such articles as wheat and black flour, meat, potatoes and other vegetables
were reasonably low until the spring 1923, when there was a very considerable
advance.

Table 1

December Prices (rubles)	Simbirsk.	Kharkov.
Black flour..	240,000($_1$)	700,000 per funt($_2$)
White flour	1,400,000	
Beef..	2,000,000	3,500,000 per funt
Potatoes	90,000	300,000 per funt
Butter	5,000,000	8,000,000 per funt
Sugar.	5,000,000	

As the average wage at this time ran roughly between 200 millions and
400 millions, with or without paiok, individuals were able to secure a sufficient amount of these essentials to cover their needs.

Wages especially of the intelligent classes, as clerks, school-teach-
ers, professional men, et cetera, have recently been very materially increased,
but they remain extremely low as compared with the great increase in the
cost of living, for under the new economic policy, individuals must pay for
rent and light as well as exceedingly high taxes. The cost of clothing,
shoes and other manufactured articles were beyond the average means even at
the present time, and the people had to augment their scanty incomes by selling anything they could to meet ordinary living expenses.

The average Russian has learned during years of want to get along
with few essentials and none of the luxuries of life. However, the constant
struggle for sufficient food to keep body and soul together has been reflected
in a very much lower vitality and a consequent high incidence of all constitutional diseases.

$_1$ Rate of exchange: 34,000,000=One dollar.
$_2$ Funt: roughly, one pound.

CHAPTER IV.

REFUGEE MOVEMENTS.

The victorious German armies, advancing into Russia and Poland during 1914 and 1916, carried out a devastating warfare and destroyed many of the cities and towns in the territory which they occupied. Kalish, on the German-Polish frontier, was destroyed immediately after its capture, and many other cities met a like fate. At the same time the Russian armies, in retreating, adopted the policy of evacuating and devastating the territory from which they withdrew. As a result, millions of inhabitants were carried back into Russia from Poland while a smaller number fled eastward from the occupied territories further north, many reaching the Volga area and some passing even into Siberia.

The various counter-revolutionary armies operating in 1919, including that of Denikin in the Ukraine, Wrangel in the Crimea, Kolchak in Eastern Russia, between the Ural Mountains and the Volga, and Youdenitch between Esthonia and Petrograd, all contributed to a considerable shifting of the population of the territories involved. The evacuation of great numbers of inhabitants from certain cities such as Petrograd added its quota to the flux. Again, considerable numbers of the civilian population were driven before the advancing and retreating armies of Russians and Poles during the military operations of 1920. After the establishment of definite frontiers in October of that year, many found themselves in an alien country.

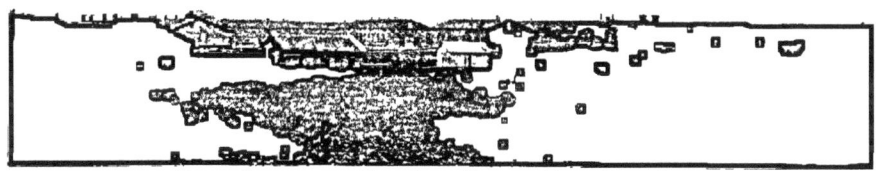

REFUGEE STATION ON THE RUSSO-POLISH BORDER AT MINSK WHITE RUSSIA
Kozvrova Refugee Camp, organized to care for the great numbers of refugees passing through the City of Minsk. A 100-bed hospital was organized and equipped at this camp, as well as a large ambulatory by the Medical Division of the A R A. A large portable disinfector was also provided to disinfect the clothing of all who passed through this point

The total number deported into Russia from Poland was approximately 3,300,000, made up of Poles, Jews, Ruthenians, White Russians and Ukrainians. Lithuanians, Esthonians, Latvians and German civilians as well as prisoners of war from German, Austrian and the Czecho-Slovak armies, materially augmented this number.

After the establishment of peace, this displaced population, desiring to return to their homes, initiated the first phase of the great refugee movement which was soon to involve tremendous numbers, made up not only of those who had previously been shifted but including many older residents of foreign lineage who wished now to escape from the Bolshevik regime, or to take residence in one of the various independent states that had been established after the war. The movement which began at once and had carried back into Poland 1,500,000 refugees up to the 1st of June, 1922, did not reach huge proportions until June and July of 1921. At that time famine was threatening

and about to cause a second movement even more extensive than that incident
to the post-war readjustment.

With the failure of crops throughout the Volga and other famine areas
in 1921, the population viewed with alarm their scanty reserves of food.
Many, living at considerable distances from transport lines and without resources, were powerless to take any steps to save themselves and their families beyond the collection of the various food substitutes such as grass,
roots, reeds, clay or what not. Others, selling their effects and cattle,
were able to augment their food resources and hoped to weather the gale.
Large numbers, undertaking to escape from the unfortunate areas, deserted
their homes and initiated the second great wave of the mass refugee movement
which involved probably 1,500,000 throughout the fall and winter of 1921 and
1922.

Travelling great distances afoot with what food they could carry,
these refugees--men, women and children--drifted into towns and cities which
had no facilities to care for them, to hospitalize the sick or even to provide
for the segregation of those suffering from infectious diseases. They crowded
the railroad stations and steamboat docks, every foot of floor space being

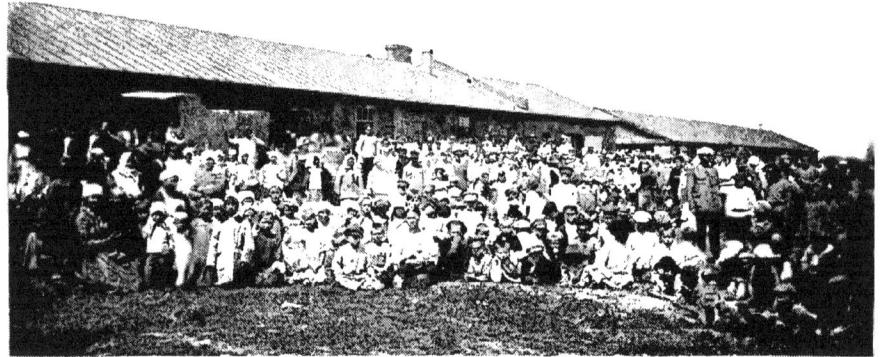

FAMINE REFUGEES AT KOZYROVA CAMP, MINSK, WHITE RUSSIA

covered. The overflow camped out upon the platforms, or sought refuge under
standing freight cars, and in the streets beneath the eaves of buildings.
As trains arrived mobs surged up, crowding coaches, box cars, the tops of
cars, as well as the ledges and projections between the wagons. Even the
couplings were at a premium. Those fortunate enough to find a place to stand
faced long journeys without protection and with little food. The greater number, however, had to return and await the uncertain arrival of other trains.
During the general confusion, families were separated and children were lost
or deserted by their parents, while many died of exposure and disease before
. . . . journey.

                        at Evacuation Measures
            . . . . shing refugees was unsystematic and poorly
. . . . 000 travelling independently and 900,000
under the direction of the government. The former seemed to have no destination in view except some indefinite point at which they hoped to be

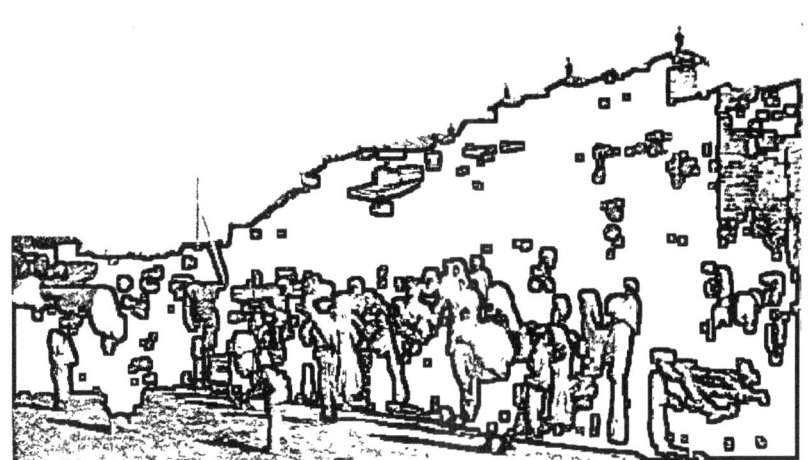

REFUGEE KITCHEN CHINESE EASTERN RAILWAY STATION CHELIABINSK WEST SIBERIA

able to obtain food. Many of them drifted toward and into Siberia, where they found little comfort, as the scanty resources of that territory had become reduced to a minimum by heavy levies made upon them. Others travelled southward to Kuban, where conditions were little better Over 30,000 Greeks, discouraged by heavy taxation, were deserting their tobacco fields and making their way toward Novorossisk in hope to get passage to Constantinople or Athens. Still others made their way beyond into Transcaucasia, while probably the largest number passed westward toward the Ukraine, Central Russia or Moscow, or northward toward Petrograd. Some of these, receiving but scant hospitality continued on as far as Archangel or Murmansk.

The evacuations carried out by the government were under control of the "Centroevac," or Central Committee for Evacuation, operating in conjunction with the various Guosdravs. Refugees were formed into echelons and transported to the more favored sections where refugee camps and distributing stations had been arranged to receive and dispose of them. Demoralized transport, shortage of fuel and breakdown of rolling stock made travel very slow. Many died en route of starvation or disease, and I saw one echelon arrive in Moscow from Kazan, where all children in several cars were found frozen to death upon arrival. There were many echelons in which over fifty per cent of the entire convoy had died previous to arrival at their various destinations.

Facilities for receiving, feeding, hospitalizing and disposing of refugees were soon overwhelmed by the tremendous numbers. For Moscow alone, Centroevac figures show 231,715 as having passed through the Lefortovo Distributing Station during the months of February, March, April and May of 1922 and, in addition, 75,000 passed through the city but were not removed from trains Upon final disposition many of the refugees found themselves in little better position than they had been in the "Famine Area." Many of the sections called upon to harbor them had no resources beyond the actual needs for their own population Consequently many of them augmented the great army of the beggar class, and finally died upon the streets

The number of refugees officially evacuated from the Famine Area by gubernias from July 1st, 1921, to January 1st, 1922 which, of course, does

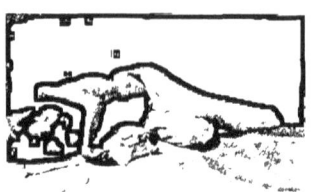

DYING ON CITY STREETS

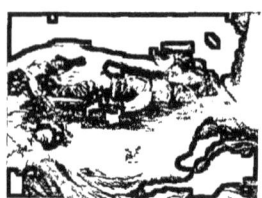

TEN DEAD IN A SINGLE CAR AS
THEY LOOKED ON ARRIVAL AT
THEIR DESTINATION

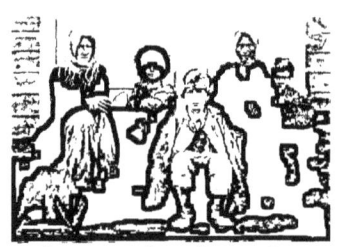

REFUGEES ON THEIR DOORSTEP JUST
BEFORE LEAVING HOME

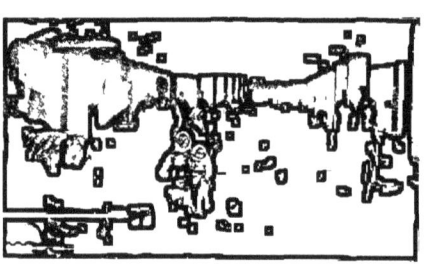

REFUGEES AT THEIR LAST CONCENTRATION
POINT IN RUSSIA

THE REFUGEE AND HIS TRAGIC FATE

not include the great numbers who fled independently, was as follows:

Table 2

Simbirsk	152,000	Tartar Republic	147,000
Samara	117,000	Saratov	104,000
Tchuvash Region	55,000	Ufa	37,000
Tzaritzin	23,000	Viatskaya	19,500
Kirghiz Republic	13,400	Astrakhan	10,200
Bashkiria	10,300	Tcheliabinsk	8,000
German Communes	2,600	Marisk region	1,000
			700,000

Refugee Routes

When the A.R.A. arrived in Russia in the fall of 1921, therefore, two great waves of refugees were sweeping the country--the first passing toward and across the western frontier, and the second made up of those who were attempting to escape from the famine areas. The great majority of the first group were destined for Poland, with smaller numbers travelling to Esthonia, Latvia, Lithuania and other points. In addition, great numbers of "bagmen" or speculators and many who had been locally displaced and were now attempting to reassemble their families, added very greatly to the transport difficulties.

86

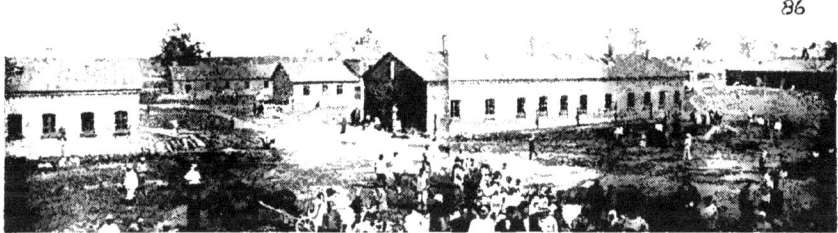

GENERAL VIEW OF KOZYROVA CAMP, MINSK, WHITE RUSSIA

The evacuations from Russia into Poland were carried out mainly through the city of Minsk, while other important evacuation points included Sebesh, Veliky-Luky, Vitebsk, Gomel, Bobrinsk and Kiev. The refugees passed through these points in train loads of box-cars, or in wagons, carrying such household goods as they could transport. Large numbers travelled afoot. The evacuation service was not well organized on the Russian side, and the institutions for disinfecting, housing and caring for the refugee and for the isolation of the infected and the treatment of the sick were entirely insufficient. As the necessary paper work in connection with repatriation was greatly delayed, and as many were eventually refused permission to leave Russia or to enter the state to which they wished to travel, these people accumulated in great numbers at evacuation stations. Their condition soon became deplorable. Health authorities of Minsk estimate that eighty per cent of this class developed typhus and in addition spread disease broadcast among the local population, and that thirty per cent died. Those whose papers were in order passed through the evacuation points with little formality. The dead were removed from trains, the seriously ill sent to hospitals. No systematized examination was made, and no disinfecting or delousing was carried out.

The refugee, therefore, carried his filth, vermin and disease with him when he crossed the border, and was responsible for large epidemics of typhus in Poland.

Conditions reached their worst during the winter of 1921-22. This induced the A.R.A. to establish, as early as possible in the spring of 1922, medical relief districts in Kiev and White Russia, which covered the most important evacuation points. All institutions in these districts were supplied and equipped rapidly. Great quantities of soap and other disinfectants were issued to all evacuating stations and, in addition, the A.R.A. imported and installed large French disinfecting cameras at six of the more important evacuation points. It also organized and completely equipped a 100-bed hospital and dispensary at Kozrova, the most important refugee camp near Minsk, organized to care for 15,000 refugees. Previous to this time there had existed no provision whatever for systematically handling them, and they camped out upon the streets or in vacant lots or herded into empty and ruined buildings.

Apparently twenty per cent of these who fled into Poland after June of 1921 had fled as famine sufferers from the Volga area. These were collected at different points throughout the Volga district and assembled into echelons. After interminable delays incident to shortage of transport, the authorities herded them into box-cars. Finally they began to make their long journey westward. We met many of these trains along the western frontier as we entered Russia. Some of them had been en route for from six weeks to three months, twenty-five to thirty persons inhabiting a single small car with little food and without any sanitary facilities. Many had died en route, but the survivors seemed happy enough as their journey had almost reached its end.

The refugee, hungry, filthy, and infested with vermin, moving across Russia uncontrolled, has probably been the greatest factor in the spread of infectious diseases, and is responsible for the high incidence of typhus and relapsing fever and other communicable diseases which persisted throughout the winter of 1921 and the spring and summer of 1922.

CHAPTER V.
EPIDEMIC DISEASES.

A glance at the attached charts, covering the disease rates for Typhus, Relapsing and Typhoid Fevers, Cholera and Smallpox for the last five years, makes evident at once that while all these diseases had previously been endemic-epidemic throughout Russia, there was a tremendous increase in the magnitude of the epidemics after the year 1918, continuing during 1919, 1920 and 1921, then gradually decreasing to almost normal Russian levels during the latter half of 1922. These preventable diseases, with the exception of typhoid fever, have been almost entirely eradicated from other civilized countries, where they are now of interest mainly from the historical point of view. In Russia, on the other hand, they remained even up to the beginning of the war in 1914 almost as prevalent as they had been previous to the discovery of their methods of transmission and prevention.

Typhus fever was always present, assuming epidemic proportions in certain localities practically every year and averaging each year over 80,000 cases during the last two decades. Relapsing fever, through less prevalent, continued in evidence, averaging 30,000 cases annually and varying from a minimum of 10,500 cases up to a maximum of 130,000 in different years. Typhoid fever was always endemic-epidemic, with fluctuations from year to year, but with a constant high incidence, the average number of cases being roughly between 100,000 and 300,000. Dysentery, equally important from the epidemiological point of view in Russia, shows an incidence curve practically paralleling the above. Failure to practice systematic revaccination as well as the lack of universal primary vaccination has provided a constantly fertile soil for smallpox infestation, and the number of recorded cases numbers well over 50,000 each year. Cholera has visited Russia practically every summer during the last century and, though the incidence has varied markedly at different periods, the recent average is little better than that which prevailed a century ago. Malaria haunts European Russia in benign forms but especially in the Volga area and the Black Sea district, while the tropical forms have always been a scourge in Southeast Russia, Transcaucasia and Daghestan. Epidemic foci of bubonic plague still occur in the sparsely populated area northeast of Astrakhan. Trachoma is epidemic especially among the Tartars of Eastern Russia, and Favus among the Jews in Western Ukraine.

While other civilized countries made great progress and took advantage of all advances in scientific medicine to protect their populations from infection and epidemics, Russia carried on a rather ineffectual warfare in her struggle against disease. She won few battles and made no conquests. With all the scourges of ancient and modern times persisting within her borders, and springing up into epidemic proportions from time to time, she remained a constant menace to all of her neighbors.

The causes which made for the unsatisfactory progress in Russia under the old regime are quite obvious. They include a woeful lack of interest on the part of the government and failure to organize an efficient health organization with the necessary authority to stamp out endemic foci and to combat epidemics as they developed. A statistical service for reporting diseases existed, but various political considerations hampered it and it could not be relied upon for accurate information. The vast extent of territory, with large areas sparsely populated by semi-civilized nomads, made control in these sections well nigh impossible. In addition, a majority of the rural population is illiterate and ignorant. They live under most primitive conditions, without sanitary facilities. A large proportion are in-

fested with lice and all homes harbor bedbugs and other vermin. As already
mentioned, medical facilities were, before the war, inadequate and the number of physicians in rural sections extremely limited. At the same time Russians are, in general, fatalists, and have a tendency to look upon the calami-
ties which befall them as inevitable visitations rather than the result of
physical conditions which are preventable and which they should struggle to
overcome.

      With the seeds of all disease scattered broadcast, and with epidemics
only too frequently existing during times of peace, it is not surprising that
with the demoralization incident to prolonged wars, revolutions and famine,
Russia should have developed the most extensive epidemics of all diseases that
have ever been recorded in history. These will now be discussed.

      It should be remembered that the medical personnel of the American
Relief Administration devoted all of their efforts to improving the conditions
of medical institutions and to reducing disease, and that notwithstanding the
fact that they were constantly surrounded by the sick, they had no opportunity to make intensive medical studies. The data given below are based
upon personal observations, conferences with leading physicians, translations
of all recent Russian medical literature, and information collected by district physicians locally in answer to questionnaires which we prepared. Those
desiring further information on epidemics in Russia are referred to the excellent reports of Professor L. Tarassevitch, published by the Health Section of
the League of Nations.

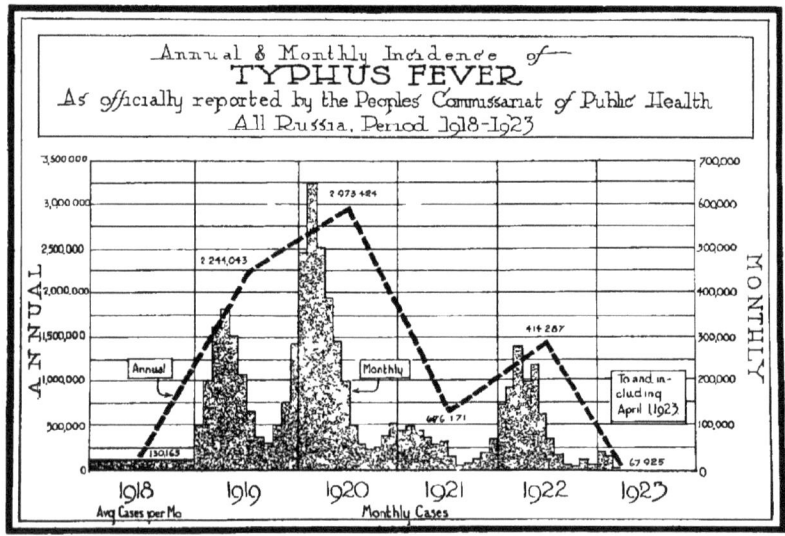

      As mentioned above the Russian Government had, previous to the war,
made little progress in her struggle against epidemics of typhus fever. The
average annual incidence of this disease, previous to 1917, was over 80,000
cases. European Russia ranking next to Egypt with an average mortality of

ninety per million of population. The annual typhus rate as officially reported from 1914 to 1923 is as follows:

Table 3

1914.... ...	86,866 cases	1919..	2,234,041 cases
1915...	89,172 "	1920.	2,973,324 "
1916..........	101,669 "	1921	685,271 "
1917......	83,793 "	1922	1,354,287 "
1918..........	130,165 "		
		Total cases	7,738,588

The official monthly incidence of the disease for the year 1919, 1920, 1921, 1922 and 1923, to date, as reported by the statistical section of the Peoples' Commissariat of Public Health is given below:

Table 4

	1919	1920	1921	1922	1923
January	101,765	491,490	89,033	151,138	36,938
February............... .	196,120	655,848	95,455	190,792	24,303
March..	318,322	503,356	87,788	277,710	6,684
April..	326,339	389,586	75,743	295,525	. ....
May....	300,991	288,426	59,450	231,747	......
June.........	215,851	199,497	62,179	126,294	. .
July.....	131,285	102,377	28,825	64,811	......
August..................	65,866	55,918	13,948	30,192	......
September...	54,099	50,339	13,494	20,670	......
October.....	93,099	52,197	19,925	18,429	. . ...
November.........	152,758	75,771	44,326	22,091	....
December...	287,548	108,619	86,005	14,888	......
	2,244,043	2,973,424	676,171	1,444,287	67,925

These figures do not by any means represent the total number of cases. It is the consensus of opinion of epidemiologists that prewar statistics for the various diseases should be doubled, in view of the fact that many cases of disease were never reported and that the statistical bureau, which collected and correlated all data, was a very ineffective organization, which deliberately aimed to prevent the true state of affairs in connection with epidemics from being known. After the revolution a complete breakdown of machinery for the collecting and recording of statistics occurred and lasted until the Commissariat of Public Health was organized in 1918, and developed its statistical department.

From a questionnaire we learned that in certain outlying sections the recorded figures represent only one-fifteenth of the actual number of cases reported between the years 1917 and 1922. Most authorities agree that the rates for this period for all parts of Russia should be multiplied by three to five, depending upon the years covered, in order to present even an approximate idea of the prevalence of these diseases. For a considerable time, large portions of European and Asiatic Russia were not under Soviet control and figures are lacking. Again, due to the shortage of physicians, it was practically impossible to secure any statistics except for the patients actually treated in hospitals, who in outlying districts represented only a small proportion of the sick. During the famine period, great numbers died in their villages or out upon the roads or in receiving homes with no medical attention whatsoever; these were therefore not included in the recorded rates. A conservative estimate of the number of cases of typhus, occurring throughout Russia from 1918 to the present time, would probably be no less than 30,000,000. Many Russian epidemiologists estimate that one-third of the total Russian population are immune at the present time, in so far as an attack of the disease confers immunity. Professor L. Tarassevitch, who had made a very thorough study of the epidemics, places the figure between a minimum of 20,000,000 and a maximum of 30,000,000 up to the year 1922. The statistics for the year 1918 are probably the least accurate, with gradual improvement during the following years as the statistical section became better organized. Figures given for the latter half of 1922 up to the present time are reasonably accurate.

Typhus During the World War

After the outbreak of the World War, a material increase of typhus and other infectious diseases occurred. However, considering that typhus is typically a disease of war, that millions of troops were mobilized and forwarded to the different fronts, and that tremendous numbers of the civilian population were driven before the advancing German armies or carried back by the retreating Russian forces and disseminated throughout all of Russia, this increase was not as great as might have been expected, and speaks rather well for the military and civilian sanitary services. The resources available were considerable at the time and they were evidently put to very effective use, especially by the Zemstvo sanitary personnel in the various areas in which the epidemics appeared. The incidence curve of the disease, however, shows a continuous increase during this time, with larger areas becoming constantly infected.

Epidemics After the Revolution.

After the Russian Revolution, conditions favoring the propagation and spread of disease became almost ideal. There was a more or less complete paralysis of all government functions during the years 1918 and 1919; large numbers of troops at the various fronts had previously deserted and made their way to their homes, uncontrolled, spreading disease en route, while during 1918 a disorderly demobilization of those remaining took place.

Industry was nationalized, trade prohibited, little or nothing was being manufactured and lack of funds and the economic blockade prevented import. Resources were becoming exhausted and food increasingly scarce.

Military events, incident to the civil wars and the various counter-revolutions played a leading role in the spread of disease. In addition to the devastation and destruction resulting from military operations, the already over-crowded cities in these areas were further congested by the armies. Authorities charged with the operation of public utilities changed frequently as the various Red, White and other armies occupied and re-occupied the cities. These services soon became demoralized, and for long periods of time, failed to function at all. Hospitals, and sanitary organizations charged with the disinfecting, delousing and bathing, also suffered. Through frequent forced requisitions of both material and personnel, many hospitals became so depleted that they were able to care for only a small percentage of cases requiring hospitalization. The epidemics of typhus, therefore, which had previously remained within reasonable limits, increased very materially in magnitude during the winter of 1918-1919; receding moderately during the summer months, it passed beyond all bounds during the winter of 1919-1920, when in February over 655,000 cases were registered in a single month. After this time a general decline began, continuing throughout the summer of 1920.

During these two years over 5,000,000 cases were officially registered. These represented only a small portion of the real numbers. The decline during 1921 coincided with peace conditions which obtained throughout Russia for the first time since the beginning of the Revolution. The Peoples' Commissar of Public Health organized a special campaign to care for the sick and to combat disease during the fall of that year and the new economic policy had, in the meantime, gone into effect. However, famine replaced war and prepared the way for a new scourge of typhus. This second epidemic wave, beginning in the fall of 1921 reached a maximum during the winter and spring of 1922 and then gradually began to decline. In all 1,444,287 cases of this disease were officially reported for the year 1922.

Conditions as regards typhus and other epidemic diseases, with the exception of malaria, are now comparatively satisfactory. In spite of the fact that registration is very much improved, and recorded cases probably represent ninety per cent of all that occurred, only 36,938 cases being recorded in January and 24,303 in February, 1923, as compared with 151,138 and 190,792 for the same months of the previous year. The statistics for March, 1923, indicated a continued satisfactory decrease.

Epidemics During the Famine

When the Medical Division of the American Relief Administration arrived in Russia on the 21st of September, 1921, cholera had almost disappeared but the number of cases of typhus were already on the increase, and we realized that a huge epidemic was inevitable during the winter. After a survey of medical conditions in the affected provinces of the Volga basin and the Ukraine, we realized the inadequacy of the resources and saw in order to accomplish a maximum amount of good the medical relief program would have to include an active campaign against these impending epidemics. Of the various preventive measures the most important at that time was an anti-typhus campaign.

The Combat of Typhus.

The A.R.A. contemplated the rehabilitation of the various bathing, delousing and disinfecting establishments in the areas of relief work, the importation, on a large scale, of bathing equipment, sanitary apparatus, disinfectants, soap and clothing to augment the above, together with the issue of general medical supplies to institutions and hospitals and thought it could adequately care for all cases of infectious disease and make early isolation possible. We consulted with government authorities as to the practicability of these measures. They approved the A.R.A. plans and referred us to their sanitary engineers with a view to working out the details.

However we soon learned that a concentrated, elaborate campaign carried out in conjunction with the government was entirely impracticable, as they lacked material resources and sufficient initiative to make cooperation effective. At the same time, we had learned from inspections that owing to the great lack of such prime necessities as fuel and water, an extensive delousing and bathing campaign among the general population was doomed to failure. In the city of Samara, the center of the famine and epidemic area at this time, the water supply, owing to leaking mains and lack of fuel, was open only one hour daily; hospitals were unheated and patients could not be deloused or bathed upon admission. None of the public bath houses, except one requisitioned for the use of the army, was operating and the disinfecting apparatus at the isolation points throughout the city, and in the hospitals could not function due either to lack of fuel or lack of repairs. Practically the same conditions existed in other famine provinces. The Tartar Republic and

-34-

the Orenburg and Ufa districts, presented an even worse picture, while Simbirsk and Saratov together with the affected famine provinces in the Ukraine,
stood from a sanitary point of view on the same plane with Samara.

The A.R.A. had therefore to use the more simple methods of disinfecting and delousing which do not require fuel. Sulphur being the most available in Russia, was requisitioned in large quantities and was soon in almost
universal use in hospitals and homes throughout the worst areas. Over 2,500,000
pounds of soap, and quantities of all other disinfectants were also imported
and distributed by the A.R.A. We took steps to rehabilitate public bath
houses, making them available for bathing the refugees and general public. A
special feature consisted of the bathing program carried out among the children fed at our kitchens in cities where bathing facilities were available.
Certain days were allotted the American Relief Administration, and the children, equipped with our towels and soap, marched to the bath houses and received a thorough cleansing, their infested clothing being in the meantime
deloused. Children received a physical inspection and those suffering from
infectious diseases sent to hospitals. This bathing of children carried out
by the American Relief Administration contributed considerably to the greatly
reduced incidence among this group.

Beneficial Effects.

The various sanitary measures initiated by the A.R.A together with
the equipping of medical institutions throughout, were important factors in
reducing disease and the magnitude of epidemics. Extended food relief extended by the A.R.A. to both adults and children enabled individuals to build
up their powers of resistance to disease, undoubtedly playing a very important
role in the decreased incidence of these diseases

Illustrative of the influence of the various measures initiated and
carried out by the medical division of the American Relief Administration the
incidence of the disease in the city of Samara, the center of the Volga famine
and epidemic area may be cited Cases of typhus per thousand of population
are shown by months, for the years 1922 and 1923:

Table 5

1922		1922 and 1923	
January......... ...	19.00	August............ . . .	.03
February..	11.70	September.	.07
March....	10.16	October. ..	.18
April....	6.20	November	.37
May	3.50	December.	28
June	1.88	January, 1923.	.30
July................	.31	February....	.22

To achieve this result in Samara the A.R.A. improved and extended
hospital facilities through liberal issues of medical supplies, hospital
clothing, disinfectants and food, so that all sick could be properly hospitalized. The two largest bath houses in town were repaired and placed in operation through the use of food packets in payment of personnel: the government
furnishing the fuel, and the A.R.A. the disinfectants, soap and towels. These
baths were open to the public without charge. In addition, American Relief
Administration ambulatories at the station exercised a strict control on all
incoming refugees. The sick were given treatment or sent to hospitals as their
condition warranted, and others bathed and deloused. Of the various preventive measures outlined above, all were due, either directly or indirectly, to
the American Relief Administration's efforts. Equally desirable results were
obtained in the other Volga provinces.

Clinical Manifestations and Complications.--In spite of the magnitude of the epidemics that have swept Russia during the past five years, and the great wealth of material available for study, the literature covering the etiology, pathology and clinical manifestations of typhus is by no means rich. This results from adverse conditions under which scientific personnel have labored, and the poverty of their institutions. However, a considerable amount of investigation concerning the etiology and pathology has been carried out, notably in the research institutes and clinics of Kharkov, Moscow and Petrograd. Interesting articles in connection with the clinical manifestations and complications appeared. Notations of a few of these may be of interest.

Among the clinical manifestations, the most interesting have been in connection with combined infections and surgical and nervous complications. Combined infections where patients suffered simultaneously with one, two or even three of the infectious diseases were not uncommon. During the demobilization from the Turkish front, considerable numbers of soldiers reached Tiflis suffering from a combination of typhus and relapsing fevers together with dry form diphtheria and most of them were in advanced stages of scurvy. These combined infections were attributed to the very bad transport facilities for the sick, soldiers being hospitalized from one disease and contracting others en route. Among the civilian population in Russia, similar infections occurred frequently. During the cholera epidemics, cases of typhus fever and cholera were seen in combination, the two diseases appearing and developing simultaneously. In a larger number of cases the symptoms of cholera appeared during the course of the typhus attack. This was evidently due to secondary infection while under treatment. In one case reported by Professors Shatiloff and Ivanoff at Kharkov, the patient recovered from a combined attack of typhus, relapsing fever and cholera.

Typhus and relapsing fever occurred at times simultaneously, the typical temperature curve of the latter disease manifesting itself upon convalescence from the typhus attack. In other cases relapsing fever symptoms developed primarily, followed by a typical course of typhus which, upon convalescence, gave way to further exacerbations of the primary infection.

Professor Shatiloff reported coincident infections of typhus fever and smallpox. In all such cases smallpox appeared primarily and typhus infection probably took place during the incubation period of the primary disease. These combined infections illustrate again the universality of infectious diseases throughout Russia.

Among the complications noted, during the typhus epidemics of past years those involving the nervous system and those requiring surgical interference were by far the most common. Since these have been very well classified in a recent report a synopsis of the same follows:

Among 7,237 cases of typhus reported by Dr. Gregori of Vologda, 887 or twelve per cent presented surgical complications. Suppurative inflammation of subcutaneous tissues with single or multiple abscesses occurred in 331 cases, pyemia in seventeen cases, generalized furunculosis in twenty-three cases, carbunculosis in three cases, suppurative lymphadenitis in twenty-five cases. There were 124 cases of parotitis, which appeared during the second or third week of the disease, and these were of the suppurative type in all but nineteen. In nine cases only was the inflammation bilateral, and of the entire number twenty-seven complicated by parotitis died. Abscess of the thyroid gland was noted four times. Gangrene of various parts of the body was observed in eighty-two cases, the parts affected being as follows: lower extremities twenty-three, skin and subcutaneous tissue twenty-nine, genital organs sixteen, intestines fourteen. Perichondritis involving the costal cartilages of the fourth, fifth, sixth and seventh ribs, generally of the suppurative type with fistula formation, occurred in fifty-three cases; suppurative inflammation of the laryngeal cartilages was noted in five and in all of them tracheotomy was done, with two deaths. A chronic spondylitis, affecting the lumbar region with temperature, pain and immobility of the affected parts frequently followed by kyphosis was noted in eight cases; osteoperiostitis and osteomyelitis were noted in eight cases, involving the tibia in five, the clavicle in two and the temporal bone in one case. A non-suppurative arthritis affecting the hip, knee and elbow joints was noted seven times. Thrombophlebitis affecting the lower extremities occurred eleven times, being three times more common on the left than the right side. A purulent cystitis occurred in five cases, orchitis without involvement of the epididymis in one case. Among the 887 cases presenting surgical complications there were 192 cases of erysipelas, among which 138 involved the face, seventeen the lower extremities, eight the upper extremities and fourteen the abdomen and breast; it involved the ears in fifteen cases, all followed by a purulent otitis. The erysipelas appeared characteristically after the crisis in all cases.

The most frequently observed nervous complications were motor excitation and irritation, paralytic tremors of the tongue, difficulty in speaking and symptoms of progressive paralysis, as well as ataxia of the lower extremities. Meningeal forms were commonly seen manifested by neuralgia, persistent headache, defects of hearing and disorders of pulse and respiration. Paralytic forms also occurred, hemiplegia and paraplegia being rare but monoplegic paralysis of individual muscle groups were more frequent and generally involved the lower extremities. Secondary disturbances such as analgesia, anesthesia, hyperesthesia, paresthesia and hypoesthesia were characteristic, as well as very severe headache which occurred in eighty per cent of the cases. Optic neuritis was uncommon but had a tendency to be followed by atrophy of the optic nerve. Tinnitus aurium and nerve deafness were very commonly observed. Psychic disturbances seem especially frequent among the sick from the intelligent classes, and psychoses, generally of a depressive type, were frequent, following the crisis. Of other complications those involving the respiratory system were most frequent: a dry bronchitis was almost invariably present, while from twenty-six to forty per cent of patients developed a bilateral catarrhal pneumonia which was, as a rule, of a mild type.

Typhus Immunity--Immunity conferred by an attack of typhus fever is almost, but not quite absolute. Dr. Fayn reports that among 1,222 cases that occurred in Rostov there was a definite history of previous attack in forty-two cases, or 3.5 per cent. Most physicians who have treated large numbers of cases report only occasional instances in which the disease recurred in the same individual, though one specialist in Moscow reports thirteen cases of recurrence among Moscow doctors alone. Answers to our questionnaire from the district physicians, which covered the experience of very many physicians in all parts of Russia, would indicate that a recurrence occurred in approximately one-half to one per cent of all cases. In no instance have we received reports of a third attack of this disease in the same individual.

Typhus Mortality.--Mortality rates of typhus in Russia, during the epidemics of the last five years, have been comparatively low, averaging for the entire period from ten per cent to twelve per cent. Previous to 1918 the average rate was seven per cent to eight per cent, but after that year, and particularly during 1920, there was an increase to between twelve per cent and fifteen per cent This was probably traceable to food shortage and lack of essential medicines needed in treatment, and the very poor condition of medical institutions. For the last year the rate has been decidedly lower; between seven per cent and ten per cent. The lowered mortality is due to the attenuation of the infecting organisms, the improvement in the nourishment of the general population and the more adequate treatment now possible as a result of the marked improvement in medical institutions.

Variations in mortality in typhus, as in all other diseases, are, of course, dependent on age, the state of nutrition of the patient, and the type of the treatment received. Among 1,194 patients, all soldiers in the Red Army and for the most part in favorable age groups, well nourished and receiving proper treatment, the average mortality was four and one-third per cent. These patients were classified as to age as follows:

Below 18 years of age--number of patients, 12; mortality, 0 per cent.

18 to 30 years of age--number of patients, 1,122; mortality, 3.2 per cent.

30 to 40 years of age--number of patients, 45; mortality, 18.0 per cent.

Over 40 years of age--number of patients, 15; mortality, 53.0 per cent.

As would naturally be expected, the class most subject to exposure, i.e., doctors, nurses and hospital attendants, show the highest morbidity rates, and the incidence among the medical personnel in Russia has been practically twice that prevailing among other classes. Mortality rates among the physicians rise extremely high. In the Red Army, during the years 1917-1918, sixty per cent of all doctors were stricken with the disease, with a death rate of thirty per cent. The rates were slightly lower for physicians in civil practice, averaging throughout Russia twenty-one per cent. Constant exposure, of course, explains the high incidence of disease among the medical profession. The relatively higher death rate was due because physicians, as a class, were very much overworked mentally and physically, the large numbers having died leaving a heavy burden upon those who survived.

Race is thought to play a role in the mortality rates. It is interesting to note that the average mortality in Moscow in 1921 among Russians was 11.2 per cent and among Jews 7.4 per cent; in Odessa the contrast is even more striking--among Russians the mortality was 13.1 per cent and among Jews 5.6 per cent.

Sex seems to exert an influence upon the mortality rate; the death rate among women appears to be considerably lower than among men.

The relative incidence of the disease among children is less than half of that prevailing among adults. Among 47,333 reported cases of typhus in Petrograd, 6,291 or 13.3 per cent., were among children up to and including the age of fifteen. Of 40,296 cases reported from Odessa, 6,386 cases, or 15.8 per cent occurred in the same age group. Children in these age groups constitute thirty-eight per cent of the total Russian population.

The average mortality among 6,386 children, up to and including the age of fourteen, as reported by Fedorov of Odessa, was 1.7 per cent, and classified according to age groups as follows:

0 to 1 year--number of cases, 46; deaths, 10; mortality. 21.74 per cent.

1 to 4 years--number of cases, 523; deaths, 21; mortality, 4.01 per cent

5 to 9 years--number of cases, 2,064; deaths, 31; mortality, 1.5 per cent

10 to 14 years--number of cases, 3,753; deaths, 44; mortality, 1.18 per cent.

RELAPSING FEVER.

The epidemiology and general course of relapsing fever epidemics occurring during the last five years, have been very similar to those of typhus. Since the conditions mentioned above, which made for the propagation and dissemination of typhus fever, affect equally this disease, it will be unnecessary to touch upon them further. Though relapsing fever has always existed in Russia, its pre-war incidence was not very great, and official figures record only approximately 30,000 cases per annum for the period of twenty-five years previous to 1917. It appeared much more frequently in cities and towns than in country districts, for though the urban population of Russia makes up only twenty per cent of the total, over sixty per cent of all cases occurred among city dwellers.

During the early years of the war, relapsing fever made great headway among the troops of the Russian Army. For the period 1914-1917, 75,429 cases were reported as contrasted with 21,093 cases of typhus fever. A corresponding increase occurred among the civil population, particularly in the sections bordering upon the fronts. In 1916, 89,034 cases were reported (Prof. Tarassevitch)--practically five times the 1914 incidence. The uncontrolled demobilization of the Army in 1918 with the return of many infected soldiers to their homes throughout Russia, introduced the infection into localities previously free from the disease. This widespread dissemination, among a large non-immune population and the fact that no active measures were taken to combat it, permitted the disease to gain rapid headway and to develop epidemics almost equal, from the point of view of numbers, to those of typhus fever. The annual incidence of relapsing fever in all Russia from 1914 to 1923 as officially reported by the Peoples' Commissariat of Public Health is as follows:

Table 6

1914. .	. . 14,900 cases	1919.	. . 225,414 cases
1915. . .	12,442 "	1920.	. 1,963,771 "
1916.	. . . . 89,034 "	1921	. 816,108 "
1917. . .	21,493 "	1922	. 1,363,791 "
1918	16,662 "		
		Total.	. . . . . 4,523,615 "

In relapsing fever as in typhus, the official registered figures for 1917-1918 have no significance. This applies to relapsing fever, even to a greater extent than to typhus as the former runs a milder course and fewer cases are hospitalized. Conservative authorities estimate its incidence from 1918 to the present time as no less than 15,000,000 cases.

It is of interest to compare the monthly rates or relapsing fever from 1919 to date. The figures given are those of the Statistical Section, Peoples' Commissariat of Public Health.

Table 7
Monthly Incidence of Relapsing Fever: 1919-1923.

	1919	1920	1921	1922	1923
January..	4,916	215,676	100,838	163,C22	37,539
February	6,181	256,021	96,536	168,904	18,200
March..	10,746	248,837	82,117	193,778	4,254
April.	7,621	208,644	63,888	146,777	......
May.. . .... .'	8,426	187,343	51,301	130,188	..
June...	10,121	148,045	53,607	142,502	......
July..	10,640	100,373	40,692	116,384	......
August..	10,721	90,043	32,694	84,931	......
September.	12,862	86,238	33,928	57,719	.. ...
October..	46,837	98,040	53,299	44,215	.. ...
November . .	36,412	138,871	91,388	32,937	......
December..	59,931	185,640	115,821	32,434	... .
Total.............	225,414	1,963,771	816,109	1,363,791	59,993

It will be noted that the number of cases reported during 1919
equalled only approximately one-tenth of the number given for typhus faver,
but that a huge epidemic developed during the winter of that year reaching
its maximum during 1920 when almost 2,000,000 cases were reported. As was
the case with typhus, the incidence decreased very markedly during 1921, but
in 1922 the figures reached an even higher number than those for typhus fever.
The disease persisted, with extremely high rates, until the fall of that year,
after which time, though the incidence was very much higher than before the
war, it began to show a very marked improvement which has continued up to
the present time.

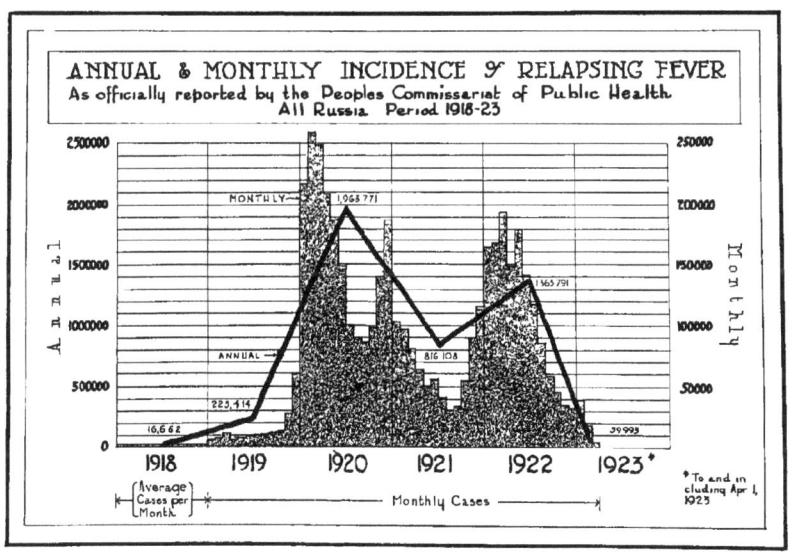

ANNUAL & MONTHLY INCIDENCE of RELAPSING FEVER
As officially reported by the Peoples Commissariat of Public Health
All Russia Period 1918-23

Transmission.--The prevailing opinion expressed in Russian literature is that the disease is transmitted by lice and bedbugs and perhaps fleas. The infection is believed to be mechanical, through scratching or by entrance of excreta, of the vermin mentioned above, into the abraded skin. Several cases are known where surgeons have been infected during the course of an operation upon a patient having this illness, and obstetricians have contracted it through cuts or punctures during operative procedures. A minority opinion holds that the disease is transmitted only by body lice. Experiments made at the Metchnikoff Institute at Odessa, would tend to confirm this opinion as the experimenters were unable to infect any other insect than the louse.

Relapsing Fever Immunity.--Though an attack of relapsing fever confers some slight temporary immunity, well authenticated cases show reinfection as early as six weeks after the primary illness. A surgeon in Samara was reinfected through a cut on his finger six weeks after recovering from a primary attack cured by neo-salvarsan. Dr. Walutsky of Samara regards the immunity as lasting for from four to six months, while Dr. Fayn of Rostov who studied the disease from this point of view, found that among 5,474 cases, there were 576 reinfections or ten and one-half per cent.

Clinical Features.--The clinical course of the disease is in general similar to that usually observed in other countries. However, certain rather interesting features have been reported.

Jaundice has been a characteristic symptom during the Russian epidemic and has in some cases been so marked that clinicians have confused the disease with epidemic jaundice. A great number of cases observed among the refugee class and diagnosed by positive blood examination, have in addition to presenting the symptoms of relapsing fever shown persistent diarrhea, choleraic in character but with negative stools. The mortality among this class has been very high.

Because of the shortage of neo-salvarsan, this drug could not be generally used in treatment of the disease and in consequence great numbers of relapses have occurred, seven and nine having been very common. Cases with as many as sixteen relapses have been reported, especially among very poorly nourished patients. While the crisis occurs as early as the third day or as late as the tenth, cases have been observed, during the recent epidemic, developing the initial crisis from the fifth to the seventh day but with subsequent relapses and exacerbations occurring at increasingly short periods In some of these the interval between relapses was reduced to one day.

Diagnosis.--Due to the shortage of competent medical personnel and laboratory facilities, a large proportion of all cases of relapsing fever, even those seen by physicians, were diagnosed exclusively by clinical symptoms. On the other hand, in the larger cities and towns a considerable amount of experimental work along the bacteriological lines was carried out. Dr. Blagoveschensky of Kazan, has developed culture media made up of boiled white of egg and normal salt solution to which horse serum is added. With these media he has succeeded in developing thirty generations of spirochetes.

Spirochetes are most frequently found during the third and fourth days of the paroxysms, but are rarely discovered in the peripheral blood during the early days of the disease. Out of 2,320 cases diagnosed clinically by Dr. Morokhovetz of Theodosia, spirochetes were found only in forty-six per cent of cases. Due to the small number of organisms in the peripheral circulation he adopted the following procedure. To 2cc of blood he added 3cc of one-half

-41-

per cent of sodium citrate solution, and after thorough shaking, the clear, transparent liquid above the strata of red blood cells was drawn off and centrifugated and examined for the spirochete. This procedure resulted in bringing up the number of positive cases from forty-six per cent to ninety-five per cent. In cases where the peripheral blood was negative for the spirochete, positive findings could often be obtained by blood from splenic punctures.

Dr. Levin, of Minsk, reports that in ten suspected cases where the spirochete was not found in the peripheral blood, ½cc of 1-2000 adrenalin solution was administered hypodermically; twelve hours later the organisms were found in the blood in seven cases.

Relapsing Fever Complications.--Complications ordinarily are comparatively infrequent, but owing to the undernourishment and poor physical condition of those suffering from the disease in Russia, they were by no means rare. The so-called surgical complications have predominated, occurring in approximately two per cent of all cases. The following were the most commonly noted: Septic infarct of the spleen, perichondritis, periostitis, gangrene of the extremities and lobes of the ears, nose and abscesses and superficial purulent foci of infection. Other complications in their order of frequency are parotitis, pneumonia, arthritis, myocarditis and iritis.

Combined Infections.--In connection with relapsing fever as with typhus, many cases of coincident infection with other communicable diseases were reported. The combined infection of typhus and relapsing fever has already been noted under typhus fever, while other combined infections included relapsing fever and cholera, and especially relapsing fever and paratyphoid.

Mortality.--The usual mortality in uncomplicated relapsing fever in pre-war times varied between one and a half and two per cent, this rate being average for well nourished individuals, who were treated with the various specific arsenicals.

As a result of the prevailing undernourishment among the refugee class, who were most frequently affected, and the shortage of specific medicines, the mortality from 1918 to 1921 was considerably higher and varied between four per cent and twelve per cent in uncomplicated cases treated symptomatically.

As a result of the better nourishment, prevailing among the general population in 1922 and 1923, and the enormous quantities of neo-salvarsan imported by the Medical Division of the American Relief Administration, which made possible proper treatment, the rate was again reduced to that of pre-war.

MALARIA.

Malaria has always been prevalent in Russia, the benign forms of the disease being reported to a greater or less extent from all sections except those bordering on the Arctic Ocean. The Turkestan, Daghestan, Transcaucasian and Kuban regions and the areas along the lower Volga have always served as natural source of the tropical variety of the disease. Epidemics in these sections, as well as in the Don Basin and the territory bordering the Black Sea recurred constantly.

As an index of the prevalence of malaria during the past, statistics of the Russian army may be cited: In the '40's and '50's the disease wiped out whole garrisons along the Black Sea coast in the course of a year or two. At military posts in Daghestan, along the Caspian Sea, ninety-four per cent of the original garrison died in the course of three years' service. During the last thirty-five years a great decrease has occurred as a result of better methods for combating the infection.

During the latter years of the war, and especially following the chaos prevailing in Russia after the Revolution in 1917, a marked relaxation in the various prophylactic measures previously taken against malaria occurred. As a direct result of revolution, civil war and famine, there followed a tremendous increase in the incidence of this disease. Infected soldiers, deserting or demobilized from the Turkish fronts, and, at a later period, famine refugees migrating from malarial sections, carried the infection with them and disseminated all forms of the disease, including tropical malaria, more or less generally throughout European Russia. At the same time, shortage of quinine made it impossible to treat the sick and a great increase in the number of chronic cases rapidly developed. Malaria has, therefore, become the most important disease in Russia from an epidemiological point of view and is extremely prevalent in areas even as far north as Archangel and Vologda, where it was practically unknown in pre-war days. Heretofore the disease was limited to the tertian variety, except in Transcaucasia, Daghestan, Turkestan and the surrounding districts, but aestivo-autumnal and mixed forms are now common enough in all sections, and in many areas make up a large proportion of all cases. Though all of European Russia is at present involved, the centers of the heaviest incidence are the Caucasus, Turkestan, Daghestan and sections adjacent to the course of the Volga and Don rivers. The greatest reservoirs of infection remain, as heretofore, Turkestan and the Caucasus. Over 1,600,000 cases were reported in 1922, but these figures represent only a small percentage of the actual number of the sick. According to Dr. Zeleneff, Chief of the Malarial Division of the Medical Department of the Red Army, all military personnel from the Kuban-Black Sea provinces and Caucasus were infected during the year 1922, with a mortality of from three to twenty per cent.

Throughout the Volga provinces malaria has greatly increased and the proportion of malignant cases is very much higher than formerly, especially in Astrakhan, Saratov, Samara, the German Labor Communes and the Tartar Republic, and as all of these are included in our medical relief districts we will discuss them in more detail. It should be remembered, however, that the number of cases reported for the various sections represent approximately only one-fourth or less of the entire incidence of the disease.

In Astrakhan 80,000 cases were registered in 1921--fifty-seven per cent being of the aestivo-autumnal type

In the German Labor Communes, in 1922, there were 42,000 cases reported, an incidence of ninety-two per thousand of population, as contrasted with 47.9 per thousand during 1913. The aestivo-autumnal type represented twenty-three per cent of cases.

In Saratov, in 1922, 97,010 cases were reported, the highest incidence being in September. A commission studying this disease in Novouzensk and Dergatchee found sixty-five to seventy per cent of the entire population infected, while in some villages all the inhabitants were suffering from the disease. The aestivo-autumnal type made up eighty per cent of the cases--ten per cent being of the comatose form, while during the previous year only twenty-six per cent of those examined had been of the tropical variety.

In Simbirsk in 1920, 45,987 cases were reported; in 1921, 42,280, and in 1922, 69,780 cases of malaria were reported.

In the city of Samara, with a population of 175,000, 63,807 cases were registered in 1921, as compared with only 45,914 cases in the entire gubernia in 1914. In 1922, among a population of 2,600,000 in the entire gubernia, it is estimated that there were 300,000 cases of this disease. Malarial companies, organized by the American Relief Administration, Medical Division, made a survey recently of numerous towns along the Volga River and its estuaries. Their examinations revealed sixty to seventy per cent of the entire population of these towns infected, the average "Ross Index," being two and a half to three.

In the Tartar Republic malaria has always been prevalent, but in prewar days the incidence was never alarming, and obstinate and malignant forms of the disease seldom appeared. However, during 1919, a marked change occurred and the number of cases increased by one hundred per cent. Eighty per cent of the entire number were of the aestivo-autumnal type. Formerly malaria appeared very rarely during winter, but as no quinine has been available in recent years, the number of cases of the chronic form have increased to an alarming extent. The reported incidence for 1921 and 1922—63,079 and 55,811 —represent one-fifth of the actual number suffering from this disease.

In Turkestan malaria was so prevalent in the Steppe regions in 1921 that whole villages died out and railroad travel was suspended, 201,000 cases being registered.

In Daghestan 190,000 cases of malaria were reported in 1922.

In the Caucasus 300,000 cases were reported last year from the autonomous Georgian Republic, whereas the pre-war morbidity was 250,000. In one of the suburbs of Tiflis, Surbatolo, with 6,000 population, 5,179 cases were reported in 1921. In the Republic of Azerbaijan thirty per cent of the population were said to be infected. In Baku 27,000 cases were reported in 1921 with high mortality. In Armenia fifty to ninety-two per cent of the population of different villages surrounding Erivan suffered from the disease, while in the Adjeristan region surrounding Batoum the great prevalence of the disease has led to depopulation. Railroad traffic in the Caucasus is also seriously interfered with, sixty per cent of the railroad employees being constantly on sick report with malaria.

It may be appreciated from the statistical data cited that malaria has assumed the position formerly occupied by typhus as the prevailing epidemic.

Due to the fact that this wide prevalence of malaria presented one of the most important problems confronting the People's Commissariat of Public Health, a malarial commission was organized in 1921 to combat this menace. The commission organized eighteen malarial stations with laboratory facilities for purposes of diagnosis, treatment and the dissemination of information regarding malaria in the Caucasus, Turkestan and South Volga regions. While these stations accomplished some good, they could not function very satisfactorily owing to lack of sufficient funds. In 1921 the government had only 2,000 kilos of quinine available for distribution, and only limited amounts were purchased in 1922. The plans of the malarial commission also embraced anti-malarial drainage projects, oiling and educational propaganda on a rather comprehensive scale, but none of these measures could be carried out owing to lack of appropriations.

With the great increase of the disease there developed a universal demand for quinine throughout the whole of Russia. The high price of the drug and the poverty of the government, prevented official agencies from meeting more than a fraction of this demand. It devolved upon the medical division of the American Relief Administration to cover the needs as far as possible. Though we were unable to import the huge amounts of this drug that could be used to advantage, we purchased and distributed over 60,000 pounds of quinine with a money value of approximately half a million dollars.

In our district covering the Volga basin and in Southeastern Russia

where the disease is at its worst, the A.R.A. used various methods to insure
the proper distribution of the drug as well as effective treatment of the
sick. In Samara alone seven malaria companies, each consisting of a doctor-
instructor and a feldsher, were organized. The duties of these companies
were to insure proper safeguarding and issue of the quinine allocated to
their region, to instruct local doctors in the villages and in ouyezd hospitals in the technique of intravenous injections; to issue instructions as to
the use of the quinine set aside for prophylactic purposes; to gather statistics of malaria and to make investigations as to necessary sanitary measures
required for eliminating the breeding places of mosquitoes. During the period May to September, 1922, 28,087 ounces of quinine were issued in Samara,
of which 15,082 ounces were distributed during the months of August and September alone. The effect of the campaign reduced the number of cases from
54,000 in August to 18,600 in September. During 1923 this province alone received 32,000 ounces of quinine.

In the Saratov district, in addition to very large issues of quinine
to all hospitals and ambulatories, the American Relief Administration equipped
three malaria companies for special work in the Uralsk territory, east of the
Volga, where the limited medical personnel were unable to handle the situation and where the disease was extremely prevalent and attended by high mortality. Intravenous treatment with quinine hydrochloride was encouraged and
very extensively used with excellent results, not only in curing the disease
but in effecting a great economy of quinine. In the Rostov district, in addition to the supplying of all institutions, malaria dispensaries were organized, where the disease was treated by oral, intermuscular and intravenous
methods. During the month of September, 1922, 32,000 patients were treated
in the railroad hospitals and ambulatories alone in this district with American Relief Administration quinine. Toward the close of operations we distributed approximately 200 pounds of quinine in badly infected areas, not covered by our regular relief districts.

Very little work is being done by the government at the present time
in eradicating breeding places of mosquitoes, but considerable improvement in
the sanitary conditions in the various cities and towns may have some effect.
Intensive drainage, oiling and other sanitary measures are either lacking or
purely local. The government took no obvious steps to increase quinine supplies for proper treatment of the infected. It seems improbable that any
great improvement in the malaria situation is to be anticipated in the next
few years.

TUBERCULOSIS.

A systematized struggle against tuberculosis has been carried out in
Russia during the last twenty years, mainly through the agencies of anti-
tuberculosis societies, which sprang up in the various cities and towns, and
which were consolidated in 1909, into an organization called the National Russian League. This league received no assistance from the government, but depended entirely upon private donations. However, thanks to effective administration it soon gained a great moral influence upon Russian society. The
league and its plan of work corresponded to the National Tuberculosis Association of America. Its fundamental feature was the dispensary, which kept
records of the tuberculosis patients in the region, and rendered advice and
medical assistance to them through ambulatories, as well as at their homes.
Sanataria, homes and summer colonies were organized to augment the work of
these dispensaries.

The anti-tuberculosis movement made rapid progress. Within five years, the league had grown to 157 sections, covering all of Russia, and fifty-eight medical societies had become members. An annual conference of specialists was held, an official journal published, and a great deal of anti-tuberculosis propaganda was disseminated through the public press and by popular brochures and lectures. The Executive Committee of the League founded a library and museum in Moscow and organized ambulatory museums to instruct people in distant provinces. Though this league made the struggle against tuberculosis very popular throughout Russia, shortage of funds and lack of government support limited its work.

The outbreak of the World War very much reduced activities of the League. After the revolution it passed practically out of existence. However, tuberculosis, as an essentially social disease, began very soon to engage the attention of the Revolutionary Government, and the burden of the struggle against the disease now devolved upon the State. As Narcomzdrav announced, "The health of the people should be in the hands of the people themselves." A grandiose plan for the struggle was minutely elaborated by the government. The Central Bureau was established in the Commissariat of Public Health (Narcomzdrav) with numerous provincial branches. Many new sanitariums and colonies were opened in requisitioned properties and palaces. But the interest and initiative and efficiency which characterized the activities of the members of the former League, was lacking among the personnel of this governmental machine. War had scattered the workers of the league, especially physicians, and their places were now taken by individuals who, though inspired by the highest of revolutionary ideals, were frequently entirely ignorant concerning tuberculosis. This, together with the economic catastrophe of recent years, has prevented the realization of the grandiose projects outlined by the government.

The central government found itself without funds to carry out a wide anti-tuberculosis campaign. Special institutions for the treatment of the disease began to close and the number of beds for the treatment of this class of patients fell off greatly throughout all of Russia. Interest on the part of the general population, struggling for a bare existence and riddled by vast epidemics of typhus, relapsing fever and cholera, ebbed to a minimum. The Russian mind is cultured, scientific and intellectual, but idealistic and illogical. Russians have a tendency to meet a situation with unending conferences, giving birth, after much delay, to grandiose plans with little reference to available facilities and resources for executing them and with no consideration for the time element. Emergencies may come and go before any effective steps can be taken to combat them, while attack upon permanent problems is indecisive and vacillating.

The "New Economic Policy" of 1922, which withdrew the aid previously rendered by the central government to local gubernias further decreased the number of institutions. Funds available locally were insufficient to provide for their maintenance. The Central Government however continued to provide for a small number of the better, well organized hospitals and sanitariums, which will serve as a nucleus if in some future time a more advantageous financial situation should make possible the renewal of the campaign against this disease.

There are now in Russia exclusive of the Ukraine, the following institutions for the treatment of tuberculosis: dispensaries, fifty-eight; twenty-two of them having a Diagnostic Division with 412 beds.

-46-

Table 8

Children's Day Sanitariums....	17 with	415 beds
Adults' Night Sanitariums..	7 with	180 beds
Adults' Day Sanitariums	3 with	40 beds
Sanitariums--		
For Pulmonary Tuberculosis, Adults.. .. .	50 with	2,647 beds
For Pulmonary Tuberculosis, Adults (Summer). .	10 with	1,140 beds
For Pulmonary Tuberculosis, Children...... . .	27 with	1,820 beds
For Pulmonary Tuberculosis, Children (Summer). .	4 with	650 beds
For Bone Tuberculosis, Children.	4 with	210 beds
For Bone Tuberculosis, Adults..	3 with	200 beds
Tuberculosis Sections at General Hospitals . ..	12 with	950 beds
Luposoriums......	2 with	160 beds
Total	139 with	8,412 beds

The Central Government provides funds for thirty-four Dispensaries with 2,200 beds and forty-one Sanitariums with 1,885 beds.

There has recently developed an increased interest in anti-tuberculosis work, and an attempt is being made to provide one well organized sanitarium or dispensary in each gubernia, which may serve as a model for other institutions. The Narcomzdrav has four model sanitariums around Moscow--one for children with pulmonary tuberculosis, one for children with bone tuberculosis and two for adults with pulmonary tuberculosis. The Narcomzdrav is in addition conducting courses for the instruction of medical personnel and editing a tuberculosis journal. During the year 1922, the first chair for tuberculosis was opened at the Moscow University, a State Tuberculosis Institute was founded in Moscow, and other tuberculosis institutions organized in Petrograd, Kharkov and Krasnodar. Popular literature is also being distributed and lectures are given with a view to interesting the populace on questions connected with tuberculosis.

The "Russian League" organized a "Tuberculosis Day," a "Daisy Day" to popularize the struggle against tuberculosis, and at the same time, to raise funds for carrying out the work by the sale of the White Daisy--the emblem of the All Russian League. During 1922, the Narcomzdrav patterned upon the above "Three Anti-Tuberculosis Days" not only for the collection of funds for anti-tuberculosis work, but to spread political propaganda as well, as it was pointed out that--the struggle against tuberculosis, a worker's disease, could succeed only upon the annihilation of capitalism, which oppresses the workers and is the social cause of tuberculosis in the country. In addition to voluntary and semi-voluntary collections in public places, supplementary taxes on theatre tickets, car-tickets, et cetera, a percentage was withdrawn from wages and salaries to augment the fund, so that a large amount was raised. This movement had considerable educational value and some of the funds, at least, are used in building and increasing the number of dispensaries and hospitals and in improving equipment.

During the spring of 1922 the "All Russian Anti-Tuberculosis Conference" held its first session since the beginning of the present regime, and devised plans for the Government's Tuberculosis Campaign. Features proposed in connection with this campaign include--a struggle against tuberculosis in children, and in the army, improvement in prophylactic and medico-diagnostic work of dispensaries, improved training for medical personnel, plans to initiate more active work in the gubernias, and the formation of a private Russian association for combating tuberculosis.

Though considerable anti-tuberculosis work is being carried out and plans sufficient to treat all the tuberculosis cases in Russia have been formulated, the resources for this work are extremely limited. The disease will continue to decimate the population of Russia for many years to come.

Prevalence of Tuberculosis in Russia.

The diagnosis of any except the most frank cases of tuberculosis offers therefore the greatest difficulty and recent statistics for this disease are practically worthless except those for the larger cities where trained personnel is available, and where the collection and correlation of data is practicable.

The pre-revolution official figures are interesting, for in spite of the fact that they do not represent the actual incidence of the disease, they do demonstrate that tuberculosis has been constantly on the increase during the last decade.

Table 9

Absolute number of cases and mortality rate per 100,000 inhabitants:

1909	....	614,743	44.2	1912.	.. .	775,122	53 0
1910.	.	621,143	44.1	1913... ...		828,817	55.3
1911.......		676,602	47.3	1919*.	.....	1,044,556	69.4

Mortality rates for Petrograd:
Deaths per 10,000 inhabitants -

1909-1913....	.. . . .	34.6	1918.	... .	37
1914..............	. ...	34.2	1919..	....	40.3
1915	... .	36.7	1920.	....	51
1916..	. . . .	36.2	1921...		36
1917........		35.8			

We note a progressive increase in the disease up to and including 1920, but a decided decrease during 1921. This is probably due to the fact that many of those weakened by tuberculosis infection, had succumbed to some acute infectious epidemic disease or other intercurrent infection. It must be remembered, that from five to fifteen million persons contracted typhus fever during 1920-1921. A comparison of the mortality rates for tuberculosis and the acute infectious diseases, occurring in Moscow, during the decade of 1912-1921, demonstrates the fact that a larger number of persons succumbed from tuberculosis than from all other diseases combined.

Table 10

Total number of deaths in Moscow city from following diseases:

General Tuberculosis...........	41,724	Diphtheria....	4,513
Pulmonary Tuberculosis. ..	35,214	Typhoid Fever	4,004
Typhus Fever.......	19,025	Smallpox..	3,550
Dysentery..	10,659	Erysipelas...	2,609
Measles.	6,872	Recurrent Fever.. .. .	2,102
Scarlet Fever	6,109	Undefined Typhus	1,136

No attempt was made to register cases of tuberculosis, and no data available for estimating the actual number of cases in Russia. Even mortality statistics for the last two years are unobtainable. Reports, however, from all of our districts indicate that the disease has increased at an alarming rate during the last few years and that its incidence at the present time is probably double that of pre-war. The number of cases registered in the ambulatories of Odessa in 1913 was 10,325, while in 1920 the number had increased to 18,788. Unofficial reports estimate the number of cases in that city at the present time at 30,000 with approximately thirty per cent of this

---

*Figures incomplete as owing to the war many gubernias were not included.

number among children. The population of the city is 320,000. Physicians in Kiev report the disease as increased by one hundred per cent. Only eight to ten per cent of the diseased were admitted to hospitals and sanitariums in Kiev gubernia and yet 13,000 cases were registered in 1922. In 1924 36,000 cases were registered, and this number probably represents seventy per cent of all cases   The A.R.A. District Physician of Kazan reports one-quarter of all patients applying for treatment at the Clinics of Kazan University have some form of tuberculosis. Physicians of Kharkov state that the disease in that section has increased by seventy-five per cent.

We made a survey of 2,000 children selected at random from our kitchens in Moscow. These children had been fed by the American Relief Administration for a considerable period and are in better physical condition than the average of the population. Two and one-half per cent of these children suffered from frank tuberculosis, and an additional four per cent had more or less definite symptoms suggestive of this infection.

Tuberculosis took on a much more malignant form than previously and many cases are very acute and rapidly prove fatal. Tuberculosis of the lymphatic glands was common and massive caseous degeneration of the lymphatics, which is usually seen only in children, was very frequent among adults. Acute Pneumonic Tuberculosis as well as septic forms, simulating typhoid fever, also commonly appear.

Surgical Tuberculosis.

Surgical tuberculosis has increased to a very great extent: purulent cervical lymphadenitis, tuberculosis of the long bones and of the joints, especially the knee and hip joints, as well as Potts Disease, make up a very considerable proportion of all surgical cases. Sixty per cent of all patients, treated in the Roentgen cabinets at Kiev, are afflicted with some form of bone tuberculosis. The Albee operation for tuberculosis of the spine has become extremely popular in Russia, as it offers a rapid and radical method for treating this disease. Under the present sad economic conditions, few persons have the means to pay physicians' fees and purchase the expensive apparatus required in the more conservative methods of treatment. I know one surgeon in Petrograd who has performed this operation upon two hundred and fifty patients, during the last few years, and the results which I have observed are extremely satisfactory.

The lowered resistance of the inhabitants, reduced by worry and lack of diversion, unsanitary and congested conditions, improper diet, insufficient clothing, and lack of fuel, is responsible for the increase in the incidence of tuberculosis. Peace of mind and an optimistic attitude, so essential to physical well being, are out of the question among a people who have been subjected to the hardships of years of war, revolution and terror, who have been reduced from opulence to poverty, and who have lost homes, friends and relatives and can see little hope for much improvement in the future. The extreme gloom which pervaded everything when the A.R.A. entered Russia in 1921 cleared up, but smiles and optimism were as yet scarce.

Prognosis for the future is none too bright. Economic conditions, upon which the physical state of the people is dependent, do not yet begin to approach the normal. Tuberculosis may accordingly be expected to increase rather than decrease during future years and continue to be a very serious obstacle to the physical, intellectual and economic regeneration of the race.

The American Relief Administration took all possible steps to ameliorate conditions. Tuberculosis institutions of all varieties were supplied with food for the patients as well as medicines, all varieties of hospital equipment, clothing, laboratory and X-ray supplies.

In view of the shortage of fats, the Administration imported and distributed hundreds of tons of cod-liver oil to hospitals and homes, and through its dispensaries to great numbers of individuals. This oil is everywhere in great demand and we have received very interesting reports showing great improvement of physical condition of children and increase in weight as a result of its continued use.

TRACHOMA.

While occasional cases of trachoma are reported from practically every province in Russia, this disease is most prevalent in the area between the Volga River and the Ural Mountains, being most widespread among the Tartars, Tchuvashes, Votyaks and Mordvins, inhabiting the northern part of this area, and involving the Bashkirs, Kirghizes and Kalmucks successively, but in decreasing frequency as one proceeds southwards. While Russians are also frequently affected, the contrast in the prevalence of the disease between the Russian and non-Russian groups is striking. The standard of living and sanitation in the average Russian village, while leaving much to be desired, reaches a distinctly higher plane than that prevailing in the average non-Russian village, where the population are exceedingly dirty and live very primitively. Trachoma appears frequently in the German Communes, in spite of the fact that sanitation among the German colonists is superior to that in Russian villages. The reason given for the large incidence is the widespread use of the family towel among the people.

In 1913, in Russia as a whole, twenty out of every 10,000 of the population were blind, while as a result of trachoma the incidence of blindness was ninety-five out of every 10,000 of the population in the Tartar Republic.

In a trachoma survey made in 1888 the incidence of the disease among the whole population of the provinces given below, where most cases of trachoma are reported, was as follows:

Table 11

Perm, Astrakhan, Penza and Viatka .	1.0%	Kazan (The Tartar Republic).	9.2%
		Orenburg...	2.4%
Simbirsk..	4.0%	Saratov...	4.4%
Samara.....	4.5%	Ufa....	6.9%

As a result of the increasing prevalence of the disease in the Tartar Republic in 1913, the Zemstvo appropriated sufficient funds for a trachoma survey in what now constitutes the Tartar Republic and the Tchuvash territory, and while not all cantons were surveyed, the results are interesting in revealing the progress of this infection.

Table 12

Canton	Persons Examined.	Trachoma.	Per Cent of Infection
Kosmodemiansk.......	15,456	2,601	16.8
Jadrinsk	27,248	5,557	20.4
Civilsk..	36,254	11,625	32 1
Chebokar..	22,700	12,679	55 9
Laishev	26,609	2,211	8 7
Chistopol .	34,915	7,933	22.7

The survey showed greatest incidence of the disease among the Tchuvashes, over half of those examined being infected. It should be mentioned that the Tchuvashes are even on a lower cultural level than the Tartars.

It is the opinion of competent authorities that the incidence of the disease has increased considerably since 1913, and that in villages of the Chebokar, Civilsk and Jadrinsk cantons of the Tchuvash territory seventy-five to eighty per cent of the inhabitants suffer from the disease. The same can be said for the Mordvins and Bashkirs inhabiting the northern and eastern portions of the province of Samara.

This increase in the prevalence and dissemination of trachoma can be readily understood when it is appreciated that before the war there was only one oculist for every 500,000 of the population, and one institution devoted to the treatment of eye diseases for every 571,000 of the inhabitants, while practically nothing was done in the way of trachoma prevention and treatment. This condition has not been bettered since the revolution. In the city of Kazan, the center of an area containing five million people, there is now a clinic for eye diseases at the University of Kazan, and a section of the Lenin Institute is devoted to eye conditions. The bed capacity of the two institutions for this class of cases totals exactly sixty beds.

Combat of Trachoma

In November, 1921, the American Relief Administration, in cooperation with the local board of health, organized at Kazan an institution for the study and treatment of trachoma. This institution has forty beds for trachoma patients. It gives systematic courses of instruction in the treatment of the disease for physicians who wish to avail themselves of the opportunity. A great difficulty in getting competent doctors interested in trachoma work is the ignorance and superstition prevailing among the people inhabiting these villages. Hard conditions of life and privations that have to be undergone in living among them present a serious obstacle.

In view of the great incidence of trachoma and other eye diseases in the Kazan area, the A.R.A. District Physician made a complete survey of the situation An intensive campaign against this disease, which is producing widespread blindness, might well be undertaken by any philanthropic organization desiring to carry out constructive work in Russia. Great numbers of eye instruments and supplies have been concentrated in this district and issued by our District Physician. In Samara, in order to afford relief to the infected villages of that province, several traveling companies each composed of a competent oculist and feldsher were organized by the medical division of the American Relief Administration, and sent with the necessary equipment to furnish emergency and operative treatment to infected areas. The companies sent cases requiring serious operations to the eye department of the Buguruslan City Hospital, where a competent oculist had charge.

This work accomplished a vast amount of good and further anti-trachoma work in the future will probably be developed along these lines.

BUBONIC PLAGUE.

In recent years plague has constantly threatened the eastern and southern borders of Russia, particularly those frontiers contiguous to Manchuria, Persia and Afghanistan. In Russia itself, sporadic cases have developed from time to time in the Kirghiz steppes, bordering on the Caspian Sea. These areas are inhabited by the Kirghiz and Kalmucks, primitive and nomadic races, who graze their herds and have no fixed places of abode. These occasional cases would constitute a serious menace to the rest of the country, were it not for the fact that the bad roads and poor communications isolate the area in question. Possibly another factor contributing to this localization was the existence of special mobile plague laboratories (established by the government in 1921) for diagnosis and inoculation. These mobile units functioned under a special laboratory at Saratov, which was engaged in producing vaccines and serum and in studying the epidemiology of the disease. An institute functioning on the same lines has been established in Irkutsk to operate on the Russian-Manchurian frontier, where sporadic cases have also been reported.

In the northern portion of Astrakhan and the Uralsk steppes the disease is propagated in the usual manner through the Siberian marmot, while in the southern portion of the Astrakhan steppes, in the sand area bordering the Caspian, where the marmot is never found, it is thought to be disseminated by the flea, through acute plague found in camels and mice.

In the steppe region from November 1917, to the spring of 1919, four small epidemics were reported, involving several hundred cases with a very high death rate, approximating ninety-four per cent in eighty-seven cases of the pneumonic type. In the interval between the spring of 1919 and August, 1920, no new cases were reported. In August, 1920, during the plague epidemic in Constantinople, the disease was imported into Batoum, a Russian port on the Black Sea. However, the threatened epidemic was liquidated in a very short time, only thirty-five cases occurring.

In August, 1921, sporadic cases again appeared in the steppe region, but the disease remained localized. It was realized, however, that these endemic foci of the disease were a source of great danger, and as a result the former anti-plague service with mobile laboratories was reestablished and placed on a working basis as outlined above.

In July, 1922, a small plague epidemic was reported in the northern part of the Kalmuck steppes, south of Tzaritzin. Largely through the efforts of the American Relief Administration, which outfitted an anti-plague organization with the necessary medicaments, disinfectants and food packages for the personnel, an expedition was immediately dispatched to the infected area. The disease was confined to two small villages and was limited to ninety-five cases, all of the Bubonic type, seventy ending fatally. In view of the occurrence of these foci of the disease in areas in which we were operating, i.e., Saratov, Tzaritzin and Astrakhan, the American Relief Administration imported 5,000 doses of Pasteur anti-plague vaccine to be used in case of emergency. However, since July, 1922, no further cases of the disease have been reported. The interesting thing in connection with plague, as observed in Russia during the past five years, is the fact that it has been possible even under prevailing conditions to control these small restricted foci of the disease.

PELLAGRA.

A small number of cases of pellagra have occurred in Odessa during recent years. In the months of May and June of 1922 a localized epidemic of the disease developed in that city. Owing to the fact that corn was used exclusively in the adult feeding program of the American Relief Administration, and many adults subsisted on this to a practical exclusion of all other food, some apprehension developed lest this outbreak might be due to the American corn ration. Investigations were made, and it was determined that a considerable proportion of those suffering from the disease had never eaten American corn. Nevertheless a commission was organized, through the efforts of Dr. W. R. Smith, District Physician, Odessa, to study the condition and treat the cases that occurred.

The total number of cases suspected of being pellagra, all of which were studied by the commission, reached sixty-five. Fifty-five of these were thoroughly investigated, and twenty-five admitted as bed patients to the American Relief Administration hospital and studied intensively. The remaining cases proved to be either not sufficiently advanced clinically to warrant hospital treatment or proved not to be pellagra. Of the twenty-five bed patients, nine were females and sixteen males, the number including nine children. A noteworthy feature in all cases was the occurrence of infectious disease previous to the appearance of symptoms of pellagra. All patients gave histories of attacks of typhus, or relapsing fever, or both, previous to developing symptoms of pellagra. Fifty per cent of all cases presented definite signs of hunger edema, and in most cases the edema appeared a few months before the pellagra manifested itself.

In most cases pellagra was manifested by erythema and diarrhea, while symptoms referable to the nervous system were observed in only the most severe cases. Mental symptoms were rare and when present were of the depressive type. Two patients, both females, complained of intense itching in the sexual organs, while in one of these this was the first symptom complained of.

Recovery was usually prompt, and this occurred even on a limited diet. The twenty-five patients hospitalized were fed almost exclusively on the contents of the American Relief Administration food packages, plus a small quantity of fresh vegetables. In the food package issue at this time corn grits replaced rice. Each patient received 2,200 calories daily in the form of bread, gruel made from corn grits, vegetable soup and a small amount of fats. After ten or twelve days of hospital treatment the dermatitis disappeared, while patients admitted with severe muscular pains and unable to move about, showed considerable improvement in the same length of time. One woman, who had dragged herself about on all fours with the greatest difficulty previous to admission, was able to walk about without the use of a stick after three weeks' treatment.

There were two deaths among twenty-five patients, both due to illnesses other than pellagra. One came to the hospital in a septic state due to neglected bed sores, incident to prolonged confinement, during spotted typhus. The other was a case of extreme exhaustion with marked hunger edema following typhus. All the others made rapid recoveries.

The commission made as extensive a study as possible of this condition in Odessa. It examined one thousand children, who during the previous winter had been fed on bread containing twenty-five per cent corn meal, provided by a Jewish relief committee. Although many of the children showed undernourishment, no cases of pellagra came to light

The observations and conclusions made by the commission may be summarized as follows·

1. The total number of cases of pellagra in Odessa did not exceed sixty-five.

2. Fifty-five of the cases studied and treated by the Commission, as far as could be ascertained, had eaten food products distributed by the American Relief Administration.

3. Five per cent of the cases had never eaten food prepared from maize.

4 Twenty-three hospital patients with definite signs of pellagra were cured on a diet containing among other foods American corn grits.

DEFICIENCY DISEASES.

The chronic state of undernutrition, universal throughout Russia recently gave rise to a great increase in the various other deficiency diseases such as rickets and scurvy. During the famine of 1921 and 1922 the number of these cases increased tremendously. At the same time hunger edema made its appearance more or less generally throughout the areas involved. While rickets prevailed to a considerable extent in Russia before the war its incidence after the famine was very greatly increased. In some districts it affected eighty per cent. of the entire child population.

Scurvy, rarely seen before the war, increased materially after 1917 and reached its maximum during the famine year of 1921, when it involved huge numbers throughout the famine areas. Over seventy-five per cent. of the population of Saratov and the Tartar Republic were reported as suffering from this disease in greater or less degree. The mortality of cases treated in hospitals mounted high, reaching a maximum of fifty per cent.

Pellagra has been discussed above.

Hunger Edema.

The typical picture presented by this disease, "swelling from hunger," as it is quite appropriately designated by the laymen, is so characteristic, that its diagnosis by the average non-medical relief worker presents little difficulty. The faces with puffed eyelids, the white waxy pallor of the skin, sometimes tinged with jaundiced yellow, the swollen feet, legs and abdomen, and the labored movements of the extremities together with the peculiar mental apathy and lethargy characterizing these individuals, once seen are not soon forgotten.

Tolstoi in his "War and Peace" described in a masterful manner the conditions which produced this condition in the Russian army in 1808, and it was probably hunger edema which Holyhausen described in Napoleon's retreat from Russia in 1812. During the Indian famine in 1912, Manson observed and described the disease designating it "epidemic dropsy," under the impression it was infectious. A number of German clinicians made a quite detailed investigation of "Edemkrankheit" during the World War particularly among the civilian population in Poland and Galicia and among occupants of the German prison camps. As a result of the blockade later in the war, the disease was quite commonly noted among the poorer classes in the larger cities. Further research ascertained its association with long continued undernutrition and also that the characteristic symptoms allow it to be described as a distinct clinical entity.

Occasional cases were reported in Russia during and following the World War, but the disease did not become widely prevalent until the fall of 1921, when the first effects of the famine made themselves manifest. Many thousands of cases of hunger edema were reported among the famine sufferers of the Volga and Ukraine.

Etiology.--While many theories have been offered as to the causation of the peculiar phenomena observed in this disease, the bulk of medical opinion in Russia is inclined to the belief that it is due to an exclusive carbohydrate diet, insufficient in calorific value, fed over a long continued period.

Symptoms.--The disease is most insidious in its onset. A history of prolonged undernutrition is obtainable in most cases, generally on an unbalanced diet and with the bulk of the insufficient food consumed composed chiefly of carbohydrate.

The early lassitude, the dislike of work and the constant desire to lie down are characteristic prodromal symptoms, and are considered as defensive symptoms on the part of the organism to save physical and mental energy.

Patients seek medical advice, as a rule, on account of the edema. This is considered one of the cardinal and most important symptoms of the disease. This symptom with polyuria without albumen, combined with bradycardia and bulimia constitute a quite characteristic clinical picture of hunger edema.

Edema.--Appears most often on the seventh or eighth day of the disease, although it may come on as late as the third or fourth week. It may appear only temporarily and then disappear to come on permanently three or four days later. The feet are always affected first. In half of the cases the face and eyelids are involved, in sixteen per cent. the arms and wrists, and in nine per cent. the abdomen and pectoral regions, while acute edema of the scrotum is quite common in children. It is painless, waxy pale, soft and dimples on pressure. The accumulation of fluid in the subcutaneous tissues sometimes reaches extensive proportions involving the arms and legs, pectoral and abdominal regions. The accumulation may aggregate twenty-five per cent. of the weight of the patient, when the general picture of anasarca is presented. The fluid is transparent, of a specific gravity 1.003--1.006 and contains albumen 1.5 to 2.5 per cent. and sodium chloride 0.40 to 0.75 per cent. The skin is very dry, the color varies from waxy pale to a yellowish white, and the mucous membranes are characteristically pale. The movements of the extremities because of the edema are slow and labored and patients are apathetic mentally, and prefer to lie down.

Polyuria.--Usually with the edema accompanying nephritis, the more marked the edema the smaller the amount of urine eliminated. The opposite condition obtains in hunger edema, the more marked edema, the larger the quantity of urine passed. The polyuria in adult patients, with the excretion of three to four litres of urine daily, in the beginning of the disease, and six to seven litres daily at the end is a characteristic symptom. Patients get up ten to twelve times a night to urinate. Urinalysis in a large series of cases reveals the following specific gravity, 1.008-1.010, no sugar, no albumen; acetone bodies and sodium chloride increased. Functional tests of the kidneys are normal as a rule. Where albumen is found, careful examination should be made to exclude Cystitis and Pyelitis.

Bradycardia.--All patients have bradycardia; in the recumbent position the pulse is forty to fifty to the minute, in some cases thirty to thirty-six. The bradycardia is looked upon as a "defensive" symptom on the part of the organism. With very slight movements or activity on the part of patient it is converted into a condition of tachycardia followed by various arrythmias. In spite of the rather moderate heart symptoms, the heart suffers very severe damage organically and cases of sudden death due to heart failure, while eating and bathing or at stool are quite common. In all cases, except those with arteriosclerosis the blood pressure is low.

Gastro-Intestinal Symptoms.--The majority of patients present marked dysenteric symptoms, but only slight gastro-intestinal symptoms are seen in some cases. Excessive pathological appetite and the extreme desire for food is quite characteristic of the disease. The demand for food is insistent, and patients if left to themselves eat quantities of food with no regard for its quality. This excessive appetite is common even in the cases with dysentery. Gastric analysis reveals lowered total and free hydrochloric acid, and lowered or total absence of pepsin and trypsin. The diarrhea frequently noted in the disease is believed to be due to intestinal indigestion as a result of the lack of these enzymes.

-55-

Other Symptoms.--Occasionally cases are seen presenting various phenomena referable to the nervous system, as parasthesias, lowered tendon re-
flexes, various trophoneuroses and hemiopia. The latter may be due to an
aggravation of the edema. Psychic symptoms are not common, but most patients
are depressed mentally.

The Blood.--The red blood cells are diminished, the count reaching as
low as 2,500,000 per cu. cc., with an average of 4,000,000 per cubic cc. In
some cases poikilocystosis is noted. The hemoglobin content is reduced sometimes to forty per cent. The average case shows sixty to seventy per cent.
with the color index usually above normal. There is frequently noted a leuco-
penia with diminished polymorphonuclear leucocytes. Some authors consider
lymphocytosis a characteristic in the blood picture, and are able to differentiate the type of edema according to the leucocytic formula. The specific
gravity of the blood and plasma is lowered. Hydremia is present in thirty per
cent. of cases, the average increase in the liquid components being ten per
cent.

CHAPTER VI

CHILD UNDERNOURISHMENT.

With large districts in Russia suffering from acute famine, and with general food shortage throughout the rest of the country, it was but natural that the state of health of the average child should be greatly affected, and undernourishment in various stages in evidence. Undernourishment is a problem which is constantly in the foreground in the United States, where food abounds for all. Of every hundred children born physically normal, eighty-three per cent. reach at maturity below the standards of health, due to disease and undernourishment in its various forms. The government and numerous private health societies are organized on a broad scale, and spend large sums in order that the public may be enlightened and improve the conditions of child health.

With only seventeen per cent. of children reaching maturity physically normal in a country with every advantage, can one estimate the alarming number of physically degenerate among 35,000,000 Russian children living through the years of food shortage and the famine of 1921-1922 and attempting to survive the scourges of disease?

Food shortage began threatening the Russian child in 1914 In 1917, with the disruptions due to the revolution this shortage was seriously felt, and after 1918 the essential elements of the diet--fat and sugar--were practically absent, especially in the larger cities. The urban population suffered the most. Monotonous consumption of dried fish, millet and inferior black bread did not permit growth and development of the children. Great numbers of parents with emaciated children standing in line for the paiok, or before the free kitchens, which issued a thin soup of fish and barley, presented a characteristic picture. Milk was practically unprocurable and its sale in the market forbidden. The government had organized stations for free distribution but these were inadequately supplied and most of the needy went without milk. Mothers with insufficient food could not nourish their infants, and babies brought into the world were doomed to malnutrition with accompanying disease and sequelae.

The famine, of course, augmented tremendously the undernourishment and starvation of the child population in famine sections.

SELECTION OF CHILDREN FOR FEEDING.

A main problem which faced the American Relief Administration upon its arrival in Russia was the selection of the children to be fed. Resources did not permit feeding the entire child population. The Administration found it necessary to adjust its methods of selection to the local needs and conditions. Large cities in famine areas, and especially those cities distant from the same, with food reserves and well organized methods of distribution, presented a different problem from small villages where the population was dying of starvation. Trained personnel were necessary, but they were not available. It was therefore expedient to secure the most intelligent and instruct them in the methods we desired to use. The A.R.A. had to immediately develop a system adaptable to the conditions of Russian life, not only from a scientific point of view, but from the political and moral as well. Because of scarcity of food and poverty of the people, the American Relief Administration had to be above reproach in selecting the children.

Among the rural population throughout the famine area the selection offered little difficulty, as the entire population in many villages faced starvation and practically all children coming within the age limits for feed-

ing were given a ration. Where needs were not so great or where the number
of rations allocated was insufficient to cover all of this class a Village
Committee selected the needy. These committees selected probably over ninety
per cent. of all children fed on the basis of superficial physical examinations
as well as upon comparative economic need of the child's family.

The selection in the larger cities of the famine areas, but especially
in centers such as Moscow, Petrograd, Kiev and Kharkov offered a more difficult problem. Weeding out had to be very carefully done.

Pelidisi System.

The American Relief Administration has conducted feeding operations
for several years throughout Europe, during which time it has been found expedient to adapt the physical examinations to a mathematical or systematized
method. For this purpose the Pelidisi system of Dr Pirquet, of Vienna, based
on the fact that a certain relationship exists between the general bodily
condition, sitting-height and the weight, and which can be expressed by a
mathematical formula, was used. The word Pelidisi is an abbreviation of several words:

> Pe--pondus decis, the tenfold weight in grams
> li--linearis
> di--divisio
> si--sidentis altitudo

The formula is expressed as follows:

$$\sqrt[3]{\frac{10 \text{ weight}}{\text{sitting height}}}$$

By means of tables computed from this formula we can insert figures
and quickly determine the nutritional condition of the child.

The results in the Pelidisi will average between eighty and 110; children with a Pelidisi number below ninety-four are undernourished, those over
ninety-five normally nourished, while those over 100 are very decidedly above
the average. Subdividing the undernourished children we can state that those
with ninety-two to ninety-four are a little exhausted, those with eighty-eight
to ninety-one much exhausted and those with less than eighty-seven are in extremely poor physical condition.

Although the Pelidisi figures gave valuable general indices as to the
nourishment of children, they could not be relied upon for the selection of
children to be fed. There is frequently a very great discrepancy between the
actual physical condition of the child and that indicated by its Pelidisi.
Children below the age of five give a much higher Pelidisi number than older
children in a corresponding state of nourishment. Accordingly, in Pelidisi of
children with a sitting height of under fifty it works to the disadvantage of the
child as it gives a higher Pelidisi number than the physical condition justi-
fies, while if the sitting height is over seventy the opposite is true. Again
the method is obviously faulty in children with the abnormal bone formations of
rickets and in those with swellings from hunger edema, conditions so common
throughout Russia. It was, therefore, necessary to amplify the results obtained by the Pelidisi test and to make a physical examination of the child
previous to its selection for feeding.

Sacratama Formula.

All children, previous to admittance to feeding kitchens in the larger
cities, received a physical examination from doctors in charge. It was found
of great advantage to express the findings of the examination by a formula.

The Sacratama formula is:

    S--stands for Sanguis (quality of the blood)
    CR--stands for Crassitude (degree of fat in the sub-cutaneous
       tissues)
    T--stands for Turgor (tension and elasticity of the skin)
    M--stands for Musculus (or condition and development of muscles)

The degree of all four points is indicated in the following rotation i, e, a, o and u:

    I--indicates excessive
    E--indicates abundant
    A--indicates normal
    O--indicates reduced
    U--indicates very much reduced.

These vowels are inserted after the consonants S, CR, T and M to form a single word which describes the physical condition of the child. The formula "Sacratama" describes a child average or normal in all respects, while on the other hand the formula "Sacrotomu" indicates the condition of the child is normal as regards blood but with reduced sub-cutaneous fat, diminished skin tension and very much reduced musculature.

Supplementing the Pelidisi with an examination of the physical condition expressed in a single word is a great aid and gives valuable data in classifying the state of nourishment of the child population.

In some of the larger cities, such as Moscow and Petrograd, the Pelidisi and Sacratama were used exclusively in primary selection of children and for the replacement of those who had reached satisfactory degrees of nourishment. In many cities, especially in the famine areas, this system was used after the emergency of acute famine had passed, while in others selections continued to be made on a basis purely of social needs and superficial physical examination. In some of the cities, where children had been selected by committees at the beginning of the operation and where at a later period a check was made by the Pelidisi and Sacratama tests, the findings of the latter confirmed in ninety per cent of cases the selections previously made by local committees. The final results of the Pelidisi and other examinations carried out in the cities of Odessa, Kiev, Kazan, Ekaterinoslav and Moscow are of considerable interest in showing the state of nourishment of the child population.

Table 13

Odessa City Pelidisi Determinations

April 25th-June 15th, 1922.

(Total number of children examined, 56,139.)

Pelidisi Number.	Percentage of the Total.	Number of Children.	Pelidisi Number.	Percentage of the Total	Number of Children.
78 } 79 }	0.4	231	87	3.3	1,860
80	0.0	12	88	5 2	2,893
81	0.1	31	89	8 4	4,706
82	0.1	42	90	11.4	6,424
83	0.2	137	91	13.7	7,689
84	0 5	249	92	14.4	8,112
85	1.0	538	93	11.8	6,629
86	1.8	1,033	94	9.9	5,540

95	6.7	3,782	1C3	0.1	41
96	4.5	2,521	104	.	27
97	3.0	1,659	105	.	22
98	1.6	893	106	...	7
99	1.0	536	107	..	2
100	0.5	285	108	..	1
101	0.3	143	109	...	1
102	0.1	82	110	...	1

Table 13A

Summary of Table 13

	Children.	Percentage.
Extensive exhaustion--Pelidisi 78-87	4,133	7.4
Exhaustion--Pelidisi 88-91	21,712	38.7
Slight exhaustion--Pelidisi 92-94	20,281	36.0
Normal--Pelidisi 95-100..	9,686	17.3
Above--Pelidisi 101-110..	327	.6
Average Pelidisi--91.9		

A careful investigation in Odessa by the American Relief Administration revealed the startling fact that fifty per cent of children below the age of four years died during the winter of 1921-1922 of starvation, exposure or disease.

Table 14

Ekaterinoslav Pelidisi Determinations.

March 1923.

Pelidisi Number.	Percentage of Total.	Pelidisi Number.	Percentage of Total.	Pelidisi Number.	Percentage of Total.	Pelidisi Number.	Percentage of Total.
80	0.15	87	2.50	94	11.75	101	0.70
81	0.05	88	3.00	95	10 08	102	0.23
82	0.17	89	6.50	96	7.50	103	0.25
83	0.16	90	7.25	97	5.65	104	0.12
84	0.30	91	11.15	98	3.50	105	0.02
85	0.63	92	12.00	99	2.25	106	0.02
86	1.00	93	12.75	100	0.30	107	0.02

Total number of children examined, 6,000.

Average Pelidisi, 92-93.

These Pelidisi tests were supplemented by Hemoglobin (Talquist Scale) estimates on 3,664 children. These findings indicated an anemic state among the child population; seven per cent of the children show a Hemoglobin of forty, 8.4 per cent show a Hemoglobin of fifty; 32.4 per cent show a Hemoglobin of sixty; twenty-seven per cent show a Hemoglobin of seventy; 15.4 per cent show a Hemoglobin of eighty and seven per cent show a Hemoglobin of ninety.

Moscow --We completed a compilation of the records of children examined for feeding in the Moscow district, selecting at random ten thousand cards of children examined during the fall of 1921 and a similar number examined during the latter half of 1922. As the results are rather striking the tables are given in detail.

Table 15
Moscow Pelidisi Determinations.

Pelidisi Number.	No. of Children 1921.	No. of Children 1922.	Per Cent. 1921.	Per Cent. 1922.
82	4	12	0.04	0.12
83	43	32	0.43	0.32
84	28	111	0.28	1.11
85	33	173	0.33	1.73
86	76	259	0.76	2.59
87	155	406	1.55	4.06
88	267	633	2.67	6.33
89	378	1,036	3.78	10.36
90	569	1,444	5.69	14.44
91	846	1,560	8.46	15.60
92	1,008	1,327	10.08	13 27
93	1,168	1,175	11.68	11.75
94	1,110	795	11.10	7.95
95	1,060	447	10.60	4.47
96	974	247	9.74	2 47
97	739	156	7.39	1.56
98	514	71	5.14	0.71
99	314	58	3.14	0.58
100	220	23	2.20	0.23
101	127	15	1.27	0.15
102	145	13	1.45	0.13
103	66	4	0.66	0.04
104	44	3	0.44	0.03
105	45	0	0.45	0.00
106 107 108 109 110	67	0	0 67	0
Total--	10,000	10,000	100.00	100.00

Table 16
Moscow Sacratama Determination.

	Sanguis.					Crassitude.			
	No. of Children 1921.	1922.	-Per Cent.- 1921.	1922.		No. of Children 1921.	1922.	-Per Cent.- 1921.	1922.
I	74	6	0.74	0.06	I	67	12	0.67	0.12
E	149	35	1.49	0.35	E	468	92	4.68	0.92
A	3,853	3,101	38.53	31.01	A	5,121	2,342	51.21	23.42
O	5,171	6,221	51.71	62.21	O	3,936	6,859	39.36	68.59
U	753	637	7.53	6.37	U	408	695	4.08	6.95
Total--	10,000	10,000	100.00	100.00	Total--	10,000	10,000	100.00	100.00

	Turgor.					Musculus.			
	No. of Children		-Per Cent.-			No. of Children		-Per Cent.-	
	1921.	1922.	1921.	1922.		1921.	1922.	1921.	1922.
I	67	21	0.67	0.21	I	63	19	0.63	0.19
E	376	98	3.76	0.98	E	331	109	3.31	1.09
A	5,550	2,875	55.50	28.75	A	6,153	4,183	61.53	41.83
O	3,661	6,082	36.61	60.82	O	3,161	5,362	31.61	53.62
U	346	924	3.46	9.24	U	292	327	2.92	3.27
Total--	10,000	10,000	100.00	100.00	Total--10,000		10,000	100.00	100.00

It will be noted that children examined during the fall of 1921 show general undernourishment with average Pelidisi between ninety-three and ninety-four; that almost sixty per cent of children showed a considerable degree of anemia, that subcutaneous fat was markedly reduced in forty-four per cent, and that turgor and musculature were reduced to a less degree.

Children who applied for feeding during the fall of 1922, were in even worse condition physically--the average Pelidisi being ninety-one. Anemia was present in sixty-nine per cent, subcutaneous fat was reduced in seventy-six per cent, turgor in seventy per cent and the musculature in fifty-seven per cent. It must be remembered that all figures refer to examinations made before feeding was begun.

The relatively poor physical condition of the children applying for feeding in 1922 is probably explained by the fact that the majority of causes making for undernourishment persisted during these years in all cities.

Improvement with feeding carried out by the American Relief Administration is indicated in the Table 17, which records the physical examination of 1,000 children when admitted, and the same reexamination after three months feeding.

The general improvement was most satisfactory; the average Pelidisi increased from ninety to ninety-two. The Sacratama examinations revealed the following: seventy per cent showed anemia on admission but only thirty-three per cent after three months feeding; seventy-seven per cent showed reduced fat upon primary examination and the number fell in the three months period to forty-seven per cent; turgor showed a like change, while the improvement in musculature proved satisfactory.

The growth of the children, as indicated by changes in the sitting and standing height, during the feeding period was quite striking. Among the 1,000 children, the standing height increased one centimeter in 407, two centimeters in 178, and three centimeters in forty-four, while 371 showed no change. A similar improvement was noted after two months feeding in Kazan, the Pelidisi increasing from ninety-three to ninety-four and the average Sacratama showing only one defect as compared with four on the primary examination.

Table 17
Second Moscow Examination.

Pelidisi.	On Admission.	After Three Months Feeding.	Per Cent on Admission.	Per Cent After Three Months Feeding.
82	1	0	0.1	0.0
83	0	0	0.0	0.0
84	5	0	0.5	0.0
85	15	2	1.5	0.2
86	18	4	1.8	0.4
87	60	25	6.0	2.5
88	101	47	10.1	4.7
89	132	119	13.2	11.9
90	171	156	17.1	15.6
91	158	164	15.8	16.4
92	132	176	13.2	17.6
93	111	132	11.1	13.2
94	38	80	3.8	8.0
95	20	46	2.0	4.6
96	13	14	1.3	1.4
97	8	10	0.8	1.0
98	4	9	0.4	0.9
99	7	7	0.7	0.7
100	1	4	0.1	0.4
101	3	3	0.3	0 3
102	1	0	0.1	0.0
103	1	1	0.1	0 1
104	0	1	0.0	0.1

Table 18
Sacratama.
Sanguis.

Degree.	On Admission.	After Three Months Feeding.	Per Cent on Admission.	Per Cent After Three Months Feeding.
I	0	0	0.0	0.0
E	1	2	0.1	0.2
A	297	669	29.7	66.9
O	613	318	61.3	31.8
U	89	11	8.9	1.1

Crassitude.

Degree.	On Admission.	After Three Months Feeding.	Per Cent on Admission.	Per Cent After Three Months Feeding.
I	0	0	0.0	0.0
E	1	6	0.1	0.6
A	231	518	23.1	51.8
O	688	474	68.8	47.4
U	80	2	8.0	0.2

Turgor.

Degree.	On Admission.	After Three Months Feeding.	Per Cent on Admission.	Per Cent After Three Months Feeding.
I	0	0	0.0	0.0
E	1	7	0.1	0.7
A	231	547	23.1	54.7
O	688	444	68.8	44.4
U	80	2	8.0	0.2

Musculus.

Degree.	On Admission.	After Three Months Feeding.	Per Cent on Admission.	Per Cent After Three Months Feeding.
I	1	0	0.1	0.0
E	2	6	0.2	0.6
A	348	687	34.8	68 7
O	606	305	60.6	30.5
U	43	2	4.3	0 2

.

PART TWO

MEDICAL AND SANITARY RELIEF

CHAPTER VII

MEDICAL PROGRAM OF THE AMERICAN RELIEF ADMINISTRATION.

Distribution of medical supplies to a famine stricken country over a territory of not less than a million square miles promised extraordinary difficulties. Development of effective working organizations to carry out relief work presented many problems and endless difficulties. Plans had to be made on a huge scale. Available resources to supply these needs were, on the other hand, extremely limited in a thoroughly demoralized country which seemed destitute of everything. Cities were congested and all buildings more or less dismantled so that offices, warehouses and quarters were obtained only with great trouble. They were made habitable only after extensive repairs.

To procure a suitable central warehouse for medical supplies in Moscow, and efficient personnel who could be trained to handle and account for them was the first and main trial. All medical supplies destined for Russia were shipped to Moscow as the central reservoir of distribution. Most of the boxes and bales could be re-shipped without actual inspection of contents, but many had to be opened and re-packed in order either to determine losses en route or to ascertain contents of containers whose markings had become obliterated. In addition even greater numbers of "mixed cases" were prepared at the central warehouse at Moscow especially of alkaloids, drugs and hospital supplies of small bulk or great value in order to equitably distribute amounts to each district. Many of the stocks were bulky and difficult to transport, others subject to freezing. All had high value and had to be continually safeguarded, to prevent pilfering. Substantial warehouses with railroad sidings and heating facilities, as well as with necessary office space, strong rooms for storing narcotics and expensive medicines, and great quantities of shelving for open-stock rooms had to be found at each center.

A thorough survey of all available warehouses in Moscow revealed nothing that would properly serve. Most warehouses were inaccessible to railroad facilities, or for one reason or another could not be heated. The local administration refused us the only building that would serve our purpose. We accordingly decided upon a warehouse for bulk supplies, adjoining the railroad, and a storehouse for open-stock and freezable drugs in the city proper. After a month was wasted in construction work in this storehouse, the aforementioned suitable building was assigned to the Medical Division. Construction work began at once, but progressed very slowly because of scarce materials such as lumber, brick, cement, etc. When a sufficient amount of material had been obtained here or there for a certain piece of work the laborers supplied by the government would go on strike, claiming their wages had not been paid. After three months' hard work, we finally succeeded in developing an establishment ideal which served admirably throughout the operation for all of our needs.

The finding or training of efficient warehousemen, clerks, accountants and storekeepers took infinite patience and perseverance. Though unemployment was general, few of the applicants had any knowledge of the English language. Those so qualified had no clerical experience or knowledge concerning medical supplies. Stenographers and typists were almost unobtainable. The Americans had to take raw human material and conduct schools of instruction to build up a satisfactory force.

Safeguarding of medical supplies and prevention of theft was from first to last a great problem. Medical supplies were not only extremely expensive in Russia but desperately needed   Such drugs as quinine, aspirin, and especially narcotics commanded a ready market and being of small bulk were difficult to safeguard. A single bottle of quinine was worth three months' pay of the average laborer. The great number of cocaine addicts in Russia made traffic in this drug extremely profitable. The Russian laborer has, besides, little respect for property and little scruples to take what he wants. He will tear the door from a freight car to secure fuel for his fire, or remove an oil immersion lens or fine adjustment screw from a microscope to provide a trinket for his child. He is adept at smashing a case in order to determine its contents; this is done by giving it a strong twist as he throws it from his shoulders, and making it strike the ground on a corner, opening the contents to view or fingers   Guards furnished by the Government were not reliable, and considerable numbers were imprisoned for theft of medical supplies. Their bayonets caused more loss than protection, for they used them to pierce barrels of cod liver oil for lubricant for their boots.

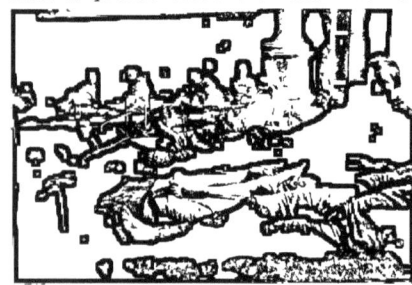 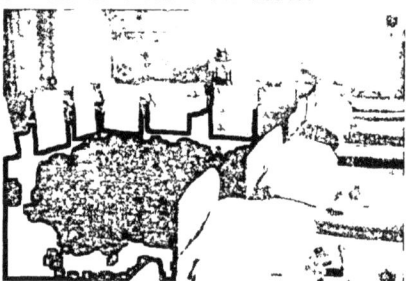

BEFORE AMERICAN AID ARRIVED   AFTER DISTRIBUTION OF AMERICAN MEDICAL SUPPLIES

RECEIVING HOME FOR WAIFS NO 1 SARATOV, RUSSIA—TYPICAL SCENES

The A.R.A. had so little control over government laborers that they were replaced as far as possible by others of the better element, who could be trained now to handle medical supplies. Reliable warehousemen and inspectors were trained to protect property and control the laborers. Furthermore, to stamp out pilferage. a search had to be made of the persons of all labor personnel before they were allowed to leave the warehouse. Those detected in theft were turned over to the Government for punishment. Our losses were insignificant when compared with the tremendous quantities of supplies handled in Moscow. Similar difficulties confronted district personnel, delaying somewhat the initiation of local relief work, but these were effectively overcome and we were able to carry out a full and rounded program in all districts.

Information.

Previous to our arrival in Russia we were without data concerning the medical situation beyond the fact that epidemics of great magnitude were sweeping over the country and that facilities for combatting them were entirely inadequate. To collect information was our first duty. We promptly learned that accurate information was as scarce as medical supplies, that statistics covering disease were inaccurate institutions. The Americans there was no reliable data concerning medie and difficult to obtain, that were undoubtedly looked upon with some suspicion when we began our work. The Slav mind could not grasp the idea of disinterested charity. Even at a later

-67-

date, when our continued assistance had brought about improved co-operation, it remained difficult to secure authentic information. We gradually learned to place our main reliance upon data collected by our own personnel or those under our control. Many provincial medical representatives, the so-called

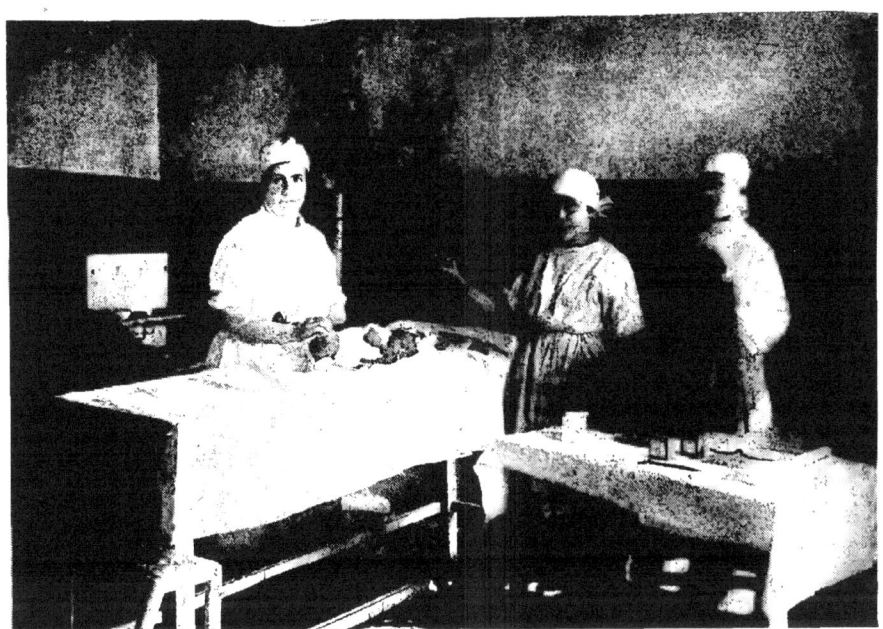

DRESSING ROOM, SARATOV UNIVERSITY CLINIC

"Commissars of Public Health," are party men without scientific training, with little medical knowledge, and with limited administrative ability. In some gubernias, druggists, feldshers and even veterinarians have charge of the public health. Russians in general are unpractical, unsystematic and rather poor administrators. Certainly, men of the type mentioned could not be relied upon for accurate observation and information. Administration of public health could not be effective under their supervision. Operations are characterized by numerous conferences, a large amount of paper work and little well directed action, while reports and returns are liable to be exaggerated, incomplete, and misleading.

To illustrate, I was given at Novorossisk a list of medical institutions in the city. This listed five hospitals and several children's homes. When we undertook a detailed survey, the Government official was able to locate only two of the hospitals listed, two others had been closed, while we later learned that the best hospital in the city was not included in the list submitted.

There was no fountain head of knowledge on which we could rely. Gov-

ernment officials at times informed us that certain commodities, urgently
needed, were not required in Russia, being on hand in sufficient amounts. As
an example, we deleted ethyl alcohol from our requisition lists when told that
its importation was not necessary because it was manufactured in Russia. We
found that though the commodity might be on hand it could not be obtained by
many institutions. Preparation of tinctures, et cetera, was impossible until we
could supply it. Numbers of drugs in great demand in America are relatively
little used in Russia, while others most desired in Russia are considered as practically without virtue at home. In addition, as the territory where we operated was extensive, there was great variation in the requirements in different sections, due to particular diseases being especially prevalent in certain
areas and also to variations in the methods of treating disease. To obviate
waste and to make supply appropriate to meet needs, it was necessary to work
slowly and base our estimates on information gained from central and local
government authorities, correlated with that secured by consultations with
medical personnel, and through personal observations of our district physicians.

     To secure accurate information American medical personnel had to make
actual inspections of institutions holding conferences with physicians in
charge, before even primary issues of supplies could be appropriately made.
Such a difficult and laborious task can be appreciated when one remembers that
we assisted approximately fifteen thousand institutions scattered over a territory almost as great as that of the United States, many of these in isolated
sections accessible only by animal transport.

     A great source of confusion in connection with our supply and ac-
counting was the fact that the authorities were constantly changing the
names of institutions as well as the streets upon which the same are located, while at the same time many were being closed, others re-opened or
upon secondary issue to a hospital it could not be identified by name or
location, while its capacity and needs were in no way similar to those existing when primary inspections and corresponding allocations were made.
This made frequent inspections necessary. "The First Soviet Hospital" at
Kiev, which changed its name five times during one year, finally adopted a
sixth name, "The October Hospital," in honor of the October revolution. Not
to unduly criticize the present regime, it must be remembered that everything
was in chaotic state and that the administration of public services is still
in a formative stage. Although an effective organization has not yet been developed, a very distinct improvement was brought about, especially in connection with personnel in charge of public services Many inefficient officials
have been removed and others have profited by experience.

Procurement, Transport and Issue of Supplies.

     The great bulk of American Red Cross supplies were purchased in Amer-
ica according to our requisitions, being shipped either direct to Riga or
Petrograd from the United States, or forwarded to these ports after trans-
shipment at Hamburg. We had been informed by Red Cross officials that we
might expect supplies within a month or six weeks after the receipt of requisitions. That estimate was entirely too optimistic; the first requisition was
submitted on September 3, 1921, before we left America, and the corresponding
shipments were not complete in Moscow until January 10, 1922, while the average time required was between three and four months with a maximum of six
months. This adverse time element was due to delays in purchasing and shipping
supplies in the United States and also due to the severity of the winter of
1921, and the blocking of northern seas by ice, making shipping very diffi-

cult for a considerable period. In addition, enormous quantities of food and U. S. Government surplus medical supplies, shipped during the late winter and early spring of 1922, taxed the capacity of all facilities making for further delays in receipt of commodities requested.

All shipments were forwarded from Russian ports to the Central Medical Warehouses at Moscow, where allocations were prepared for all districts. Transport, during the first year of our operations, was in a deplorable state. It required one month to six weeks for supplies to reach Moscow from ports, and an equal length of time to get them from Moscow to the various districts.

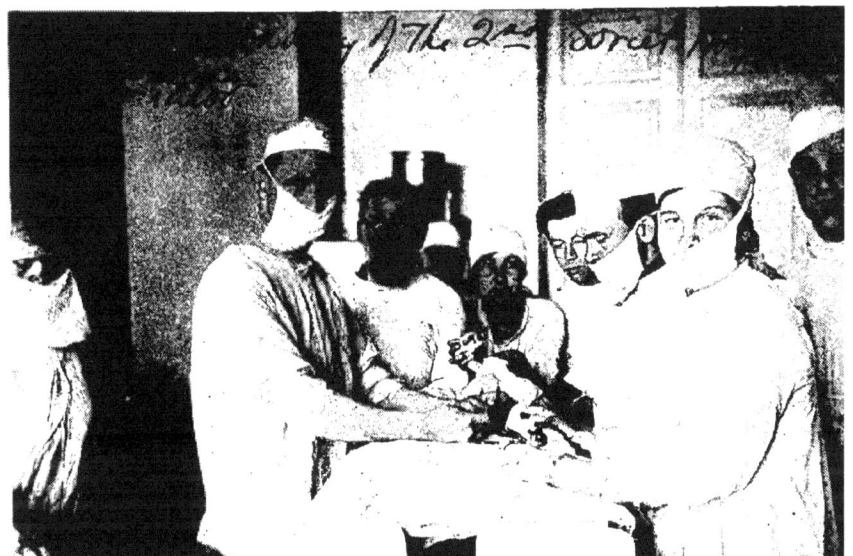

PROFESSOR RAZOUMINSKY IN HIS CLINIC, SARATOV UNIVERSITY
Thousands of such institutions only carried on by the medical supplies from America. Bandages, bedding, instruments, anæsthetics, medicines from America enabled them to do their part in relief of famine and disease.

These delays did not materially interfere with the initiation of our program, for we had been fortunate in securing from the American Red Cross stocks in Paris, a donation of approximately seven hundred thousand dollars worth of medical supplies in addition to the original gift of three million dollars. Though these stocks were not well rounded, they included quantities of essential drugs, disinfectants, surgical dressings and hospital clothing, and as they arrived in Russia very promptly by overland shipments, we were able to begin work without material delay. Development of our full program of relief was somewhat retarded, incident to delays in receipt of supplies requested, but we overcame it as far as possible by promptly making our requisitions on America, and for much larger quantities of the various items that we would have requested at the moment had shipments been more prompt.

In like manner we attempted to prevent delays in organizing the relief in the various districts by making shipments long in advance of the arrival of District Physicians from America, but we were not always successful in this. We forwarded two carloads of well rounded supplies to Tzaritzin three weeks before Dr. Cornick, the prospective District Physician, arrived in Moscow, December 15, 1921, and instructed the doctor to begin relief work at once, as all supplies would be on hand. We were accordingly quite chagrined to receive a telegram from him on January 5, 1922, requesting us to forward to Tzaritzin, by courier, a small packet of medicines for treatment of American personnel. The train of supplies was held snow-bound for a considerable time but finally arrived after an interval of seven weeks.

Though delays in the procurement and transport of supplies from the United States to various district headquarters caused constant worry and anxiety, difficulties at Moscow were insignificant compared with those of district physicians who were charged not only with distribution to institutions throughout their districts, but also with an accurate accounting for all issues made. The districts covered vast areas with few large cities but with hundreds of towns and villages, where small hospitals, ambulatories or feldsher points had to be reached. Most of the towns are isolated, as few railroads exist; many are accessible by water transport in the summer but can be reached only by sledges during winter months. Draft animals were scarce, especially during the winter of 1921, as many had died of famine or had been slaughtered for food and those remaining were weak and not in condition to handle heavy burdens. But the great need induced superhuman efforts; means of transport were somehow developed, and large quantities of supplies were distributed and accounted for during the winter of 1921. Inspection trips covering great distances, under most adverse climatic conditions and with temperature twenty to thirty degrees below zero, had to be frequently made. Days were spent en route and nights in peasant huts in constant danger of typhus and other infectious diseases. But based upon the information gained, large quantities of medical supplies were soon transported by convoys of sledges to institutions in great need of everything to treat the sick.

Government surplus stocks donated by America proved a great boon to the people of Russia but they were not an unalloyed blessing to the medical personnel who were required to handle them. We had made all preparations for their reception in Moscow and in the districts by increasing several fold the capacity of our warehouses, the central warehouse in Moscow having finally a capacity of two hundred carloads, while those in districts could accommodate from ten to twenty-five carloads each in addition to open stock rooms and assembling departments. Increased personnel, warehousemen, clerks and laborers were also employed and given a thorough course of training.

Tremendous quantities of United States Government surplus stocks and Red Cross supplies held up by shipping troubles began to arrive in June, 1922, and continued for the following three months, during which time four hundred and forty-eight carloads were received and three hundred and thirty-one were dispatched to districts. All facilities for receiving, checking, accounting and re-allocating were taxed to the limit during this period. Warehousing accommodations were at times insufficient, and stocks were stored temporarily in tents, under tarpaulins, and in available food storage warehouses. Temporary delay and some confusion occurred because invoices and packers' lists covering stocks shipped from the Atlanta Depot, by far the largest source of all Government Surplus supplies, were not properly prepared, making the identification and check of cases impossible. The difficulty was overcome by making an index of four thousand cards for the eight hundred pages of Atlanta invoices as an emergency measure, and later completed a one hundred and sixty page packers' list, with all numbers and data properly arranged. This obviated further difficulty, and we were able in the long run to identify every case received either from our invoices, or by examination of contents, where duplication of numbers or obliteration of the same from cases, made this necessary. We were also able to cover all shipments to districts by accurate invoices for all commodities shipped. These and other measures gave us at the termination of the operation, complete commodity reports for all United States Government surplus and Red Cross supplies, with substantiating receipts from beneficiaries for every item issued.

United States Government stocks contained many items in very large amounts, a considerable number of which were little known in Russia; at the same time the entire shipment was not well balanced with needs. We accordingly used the remaining Red Cross funds to round out our supply table. Coincidently we had to carry on considerable educational work, instructing local physicians in the use of drugs, with which they were not acquainted. Many preparations, such as Pill. Mistura Glycyrrhyzae Comp. and Pill. Cathartic Compound, previously practically unknown in Russia soon became popular for prescriptions of Russian physicians.

Government Cooperation.

Our relations with the Commissar of Public Health and his assistants were most cordial throughout. We kept his office constantly informed of all measures of relief being carried out, frequently seeking his advice and assistance.

On the whole we had better cooperation than other divisions of the A.R.A. in Russia. This is probably due to the fact that the physicians, with whom we dealt mainly, are of a class better educated and with greater vision than the average individual in government service, and also because our demands were small. Nevertheless, more or less interference on the part of government officials was found in each district when we began operating, and had to be overcome before satisfactory relief work could be carried out. But in only one, the sub-district of Vitebsk, was this interference systematic and continuous, inducing us to limit our assistance in this area. This interference manifested itself mainly in an attempt to secure control of our resources, evidenced in an attempt to induce us to warehouse our stocks in government warehouse, insisting that requisitions from institutions be made through them and not direct to us, and elaborating systems of distribution which would remove control from our hands. A firm stand by our personnel, as a rule, quite easily overcame such interference, although in Saratov orders were issued temporarily barring American physicians and their representatives from all institutions, due to our refusal to accept the government system of distribution.

In a few instances, as in Ufa and Odessa, our supplies were requisitioned by government officials from hospitals, after we had made distributions, but they were returned upon our demand. Peculiarly enough the question of aiding Moscow institutions was not looked upon with favor by the local authorities. In spite of the numerous requests for assistance which were being made to us daily by personnel in charge we were informed that Moscow hospitals had everything needed. Our inspections later revealed them in almost as great need as even those in the Volga area where we began operating, and our distributions to the City and Gubernia were later carried out on a very large scale without any difficulty.

On the whole, interference was local and not systematic, and in some districts hearty co-operation on the part of the government made possible a much more intensive and satisfactory program than would have been possible without their assistance.

Travel and Inspection.

The demoralized condition of transport, as well as the adverse general conditions under which we operated during the first year of our work in Russia, made tours of inspection extremely difficult and time consuming. Trips frequently required as many days as under normal conditions could have been covered in hours.

Transport of our personnel into Russia and their distribution to various districts, as well as travel within the local areas on trips of inspection and control, caused constant worry. The public coaches of trains were jammed with great masses of people travelling in every direction, congesting compartments, aisles and platforms of cars, where they sat or stood for days and nights on long journeys. Refugees and "bagmen," or speculators, formed most of the travelling public. Infested with lice and some actually suffering from infectious diseases, these menaced their fellow travellers. Most of the coaches were of the second or fourth class variety, and modern accommodations or decent sanitary conditions were non-existent. The danger of travel in public coaches was extremely great, and though a considerable number of private cars were available for American supervisors, they were insufficient to care for the American personnel. Travel by sledges in districts, with rests at night in unsanitary and infested peasants' homes, was even more dangerous than rail trips.

All of the American workers were protected by vaccinations, inoculations and all varieties of insecticides. They were instructed thoroughly concerning personal protection, but nevertheless their health occasioned constant apprehension. In spite of the great number of Americans in Russia--a maximum of approximately 200--we were fortunate that only eight of our personnel developed typhus fever, with one death. Four cases of pneumonia, two of relapsing fever and two of undetermined fever suggesting abortive typhoid, all of which terminating favorably completed the sick record of the personnel. Other organizations operating in Russia had very much higher mortality and morbidity rates, over fifty per cent of the members of the "Friends" organization developing typhus fever alone during the winter of 1921 and 1922.

Table 19
RESOURCES.

The total resources of the American Relief Administration for medical relief work in Russia were as follows:

1. An appropriation of $3,000,000 from the American Red Cross⟩
2. A donation of medical and hospital supplies and winter ⟩ $3,804,863.15
   clothing from the Paris stocks of the American Red Cross..⟩
3. The Congressional donation of Government Surplus Medical
   Supplies.... .... 4,000,000.00
   (The expenses incurred in inspecting, handling and shipping these supplies were defrayed by a gift of $500,000 from the Laura Spelman Rockefeller Memorial Foundation, $267,392.88 of which was actually used in this work)....... 267,392.88
4. Food and clothing packets for medical personnel. Three donations by Mr. William Bingham, 2nd, of Boston, Mass., to be administered by Dr. Henry Beeuwkes......... .... 95,000.00
5. Donation from the Rochester Community Chest.. .... 5,000.00
6. Donation from Dr. Henry O. Eversole....................... 5,000.00
   Total of donations.. . ...$8,177,256.03

-73-

Additional miscellaneous gifts of medicines, hospital supplies, et cetera, were received from the United States Treasury, the American Red Cross and other organizations in America, and a donation of $25,000 for food packets for physicians was administered jointly by the Joint Distribution Committee, which provided the funds, and the Medical Director of the American Relief Administration.

In addition, the Rockefeller Foundation provided medical literature in generous amounts for distribution among universities and other institutions through our organization.

The entire cost of the medical operation in Russia, exclusive of that borne by the Soviet Government under the "Riga Agreement," was paid by the American Relief Administration and included the salaries of American physicians and other medical personnel. All of the appropriation donated by the American Red Cross was, therefore, available for actual medical relief and was expended for the purchase of medical, hospital and laboratory supplies, disinfectants and sanitary equipment. These resources proved ample to carry out emergency operations on a grand scale and a considerable amount of constructive work as well.

We had feared in the fall of 1922 that it would be necessary either to secure additional funds or to curtail the work, but the very great reduction in disease in general as well as the absence of epidemics of large proportions made for a great saving in all supplies. Consequently, we were able to continue a full and rounded program in all districts up to the termination of our activities and leave institutions well stocked upon our withdrawal. In addition we made very generous donations during March, April and May of 1923 to large numbers of hospitals and dispensaries in areas not included in our relief districts.

CHAPTER VIII
PLAN AND SCOPE OF MEDICAL RELIEF

In outlining the plan and scope of the medical relief program the factors which had to be taken into consideration included the most pressing needs, the resources at hand, the local facilities available to assist in carrying out particular lines of work, and finally, the various difficulties and adverse circumstances, mentioned above, which made certain varieties of relief impracticable.

The situation to be met was briefly as follows: Epidemics of great magnitude reigned throughout Russia, while facilities for combatting the same were extremely limited, and medical institutions, though present in large numbers and generally well administered, were unable to function effectively due to shortage of all classes of medical supplies and lack of food for patients and personnel. Our aim accordingly became to employ all of our resources in improving sanitary conditions, reducing disease and relieving the poverty of medical institutions.

We strove to make our program as practical as possible and obviate loss and waste. Many measures which presented themselves for our consideration and which under ordinary circumstances might have been desirable, would have been entirely impracticable due to peculiar local conditions. We had contemplated a very extensive delousing campaign throughout the Volga Basin against the vermin-borne diseases, involving the importation of disinfectors, bathing apparatus, replacement clothing, et cetera. But we abandoned the idea when we discovered that much of the existing apparatus for bathing and delousing was not in operation because of the inertia of the authorities and due to shortage of fuel and even of water throughout the region. Hospitals at that time could not bathe even infectious patients, as water was available only for a few hours each night.

We accordingly compromised, importing a small number of disinfectors for special purposes to be used where water and fuel were available, and great quantities of soap, sulphur and other disinfectants which we issued broadcast to individual institutions. A mass inoculation campaign on the other hand, appeared practicable and successfully we carried it out since we could supply all necessary materials for conducting the work independently of local assistance. At the same time we had sufficient control, at least over the children whom we fed, to make inoculation compulsory.

We aimed to assist thousands of institutions rather than to organize a few "model institutions," as was frequently suggested, believing it wiser to place existing hospitals in a position to function rather than to supply them with models which their poverty would not permit them to imitate. Had we attempted this rather idealistic and local type of relief, much time and energy would probably have been wasted, and an effective relief program on a large scale would have been correspondingly retarded.

The program finally adopted and carried out successfully in all of our districts was as follows:

1. The supply of existing hospitals, dispensaries, feldsher points, laboratories, and other sanitary formations with all essentials necessary to carry out effective work.
2. The organization and administration of ambulatories and pharmacies where needed.
3. Assistance to homes for children, the aged, blind, et cetera.
4. Issue of food for hospital patients and inmates of homes.

5. Measures to reduce disease and improve sanitary conditions.
   Inoculation Campaign.
   Clean-Up Campaign.
   Supply of disinfectants and disinfecting apparatus.
   Improvement of water supply of cities.
   Bathing Campaigns.
6. Food and clothing relief for medical personnel.
7. Supply of medical literature to universities and other institutions.

Though inaugurated primarily to relieve an existing emergency this program included, especially towards the close of operations, a very considerable amount of reconstructive work. Our gifts included large quantities of non-expendable articles and permanent equipment such as microscope, radiographic apparatus, operating and bedside tables and all classes of enamel ware, as well as very extensive donations of all varieties of surgical apparatus, ophthalmoscopes, cystoscopes, general and special operating sets, and many other items of a permanent nature. The tremendous quantities of bedding and hospital clothing issued to institutions should cover the need for these classes of supplies for a considerable number of years to come.

Organization.

Moscow, centrally located, the seat of Government, and having direct railroad communications with all parts of Russia, was selected as the Headquarters of the American Relief Administration. For purposes of local administration, the entire area in which we operated was divided into districts, each with its own machinery for carrying out the work and with local headquarters situated in the largest city or town.

The Moscow organization included the Administrative offices and general medical warehouses. The personnel of the former consisted of the Chief of the Medical Division, a staff of three Americans and a considerable number of Russian personnel serving as interpreters, translators and clerical forces. Their duties included the general direction of all medical relief work throughout Russia. Specifically they were as follows:

1. The collection of information concerning disease conditions and medical needs.

2. Decision as to the most appropriate lines of relief to be undertaken and areas in which it should be carried out. It was intended primarily to limit medical and food relief to the Volga or so-called "Famine Area." However, we learned early during the operation that our resources would permit of a considerable extension of the work territorially and especially so after their great increase through the donation of the Government Surplus stocks. We had likewise discovered that the needs in the Ukraine, especially in the southern parts, were as great as in the Volga section and that the medical famine was more or less general throughout Russia. We therefore increased the number and size of our districts as rapidly as possible, covering primarily and most intensively those areas in most dire need and later extending more limited relief to other sections.

3. Preparation of timely requisitions for supplies to be purchased in America or abroad.

4. Accounting for supplies received in Moscow and their allocation to districts.

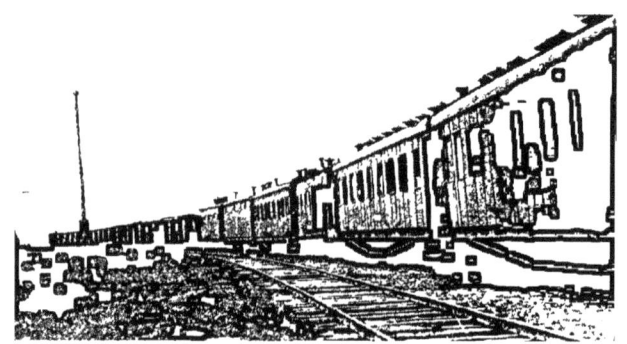

The train as it left Moscow, made up of 22 cars of medical supplies and convoy, distributing medicines and supplies to over 500 institutions in areas outside regular districts of the American Relief Administration

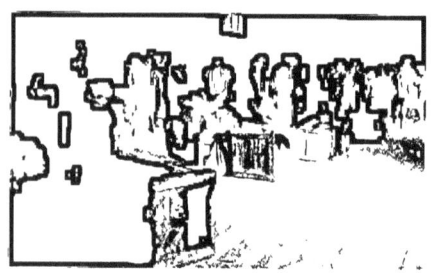

DISTRIBUTING MEDICAL SUPPLIES AT STATION AT OREL

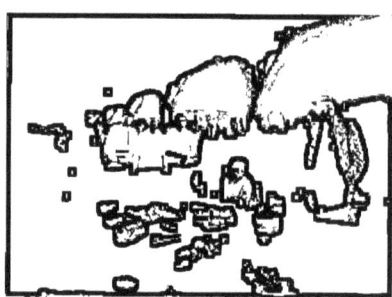

DISTRIBUTION AT RAILWAY STATION TULA

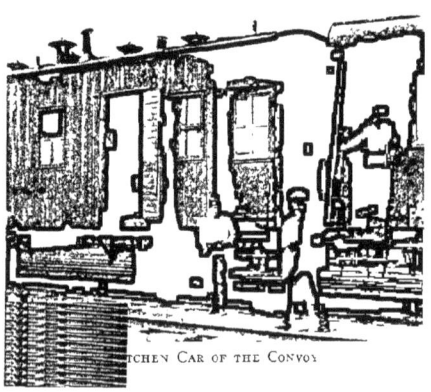

KITCHEN CAR OF THE CONVOY

AMERICAN SANITARY TRAIN NO. 1

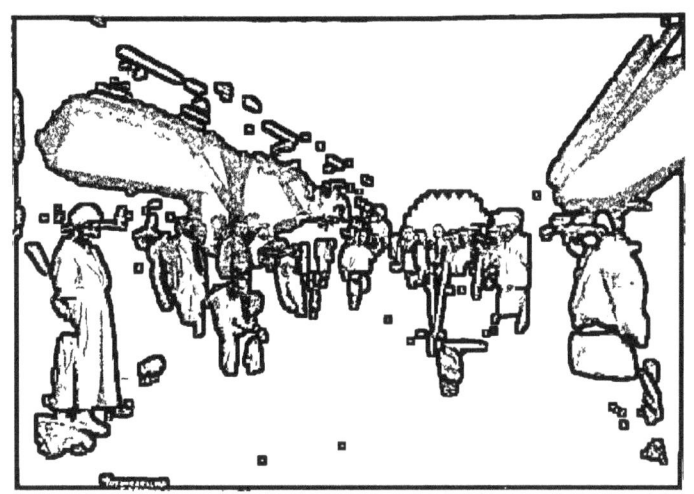

ARRIVAL OF AMERICAN MEDICAL SUPPLIES AT OREL

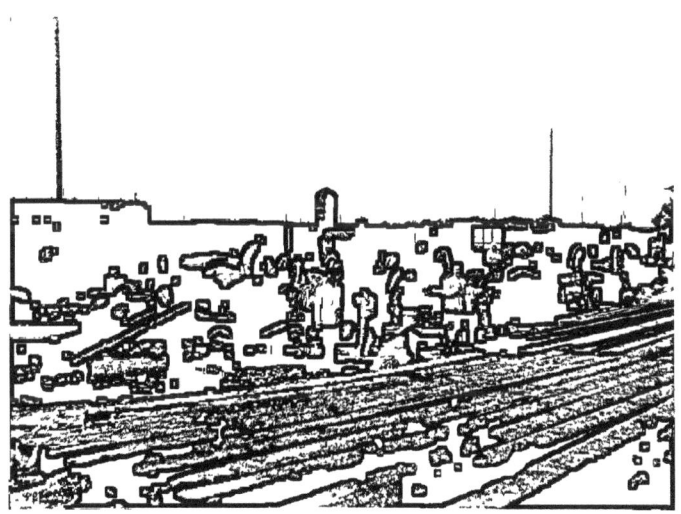

LOADING SUPPLIES FOR OUTLYING TOWNS

SANITARY TRAIN NO 1

5. Supervision of all district accounting and check of all commodity reports.

All requisitions for supplies to be purchased in America or abroad, as well as the allocations of the same to the various districts, were prepared personally by the Chief of the Medical Division of the A.R.A. Early requisitions covered only essentials in limited amounts, but as our knowledge concerning needs became more specific and after a definite policy as to the nature and extent of relief had been formulated, the number of items requested was very much amplified. At the same time maximum quantities were ordered in order to obviate loss of time from the numerous delays in purchase and shipment mentioned above. Our "Requisition No. 18" alone covered medicines and hospital supplies to a value of well over five hundred thousand dollars.

We attempted to provide all essential items and keep stocks constantly well rounded in the various districts. The Russian physicians' ideas of essentials, however, differ quite widely from those prevailing in America, and we had therefore to adopt our supply tables to their needs as we learned them. We kept constantly in touch with the supply situation in all districts, and based our requisitions on America, upon the amounts of the various items issued and expended in the past.

Permanent and semi-permanent equipment and hospital supplies were in general issued to the various districts upon a percentage basis, the percentage value given each district being based upon its size, population and the number and capacity of hospitals, homes and other institutions. Other factors such as transport facility, local cooperation or lack of the same, and relative needs were also taken into consideration. As regards medicines and expendable supplies, however, we based our allocations almost exclusively upon local needs as indicated by past issues and frequent reports from District Physicians.

The technique involved in the procurement, warehousing, issue, and accounting for medical supplies will be discussed below. It should be mentioned here, however, that all commodity reports from districts and substantiating receipts from beneficiary institutions were very thoroughly checked in our office in Moscow and all necessary corrections made previous to their being forwarded to the United States. An accurate accounting was rendered covering all medical supplies received in Russia.

6. Instruction of Personnel and Inspection, Correlation and Control of all district work.

All physicians before proceeding to duty in districts received a course of instruction in Moscow covering essential features of the work, and especially in connection with accounting and in the preparation of general and commodity reporting. Inspections of the district work were carried out as far as possible by Moscow personnel, though the difficulties of transport made this a very time consuming process. District personnel were kept constantly informed on all matters pertaining to the medical work by very numerous formal and informal circulars. District Physicians made monthly reports covering local conditions and work accomplished. These reports, including the "Form A" showing in detail the numbers and capacity of all institutions assisted, together with details as to nature and amount of assistance rendered and data concerning each institution supplied, were all correlated and consolidated in the Moscow office.

7. Preparation of Reports. Reports covering medical conditions in Russia were forwarded monthly to the United States together with consolidated

reports showing the amount of work accomplished in all districts. Commodity reports covering all shipments received in Moscow and all issues made to the various districts were also forwarded each month, while the commodity reports of districts were made at three month intervals.

       8.   Initiation of measures for the health of personnel

       9.   Care of the Sick

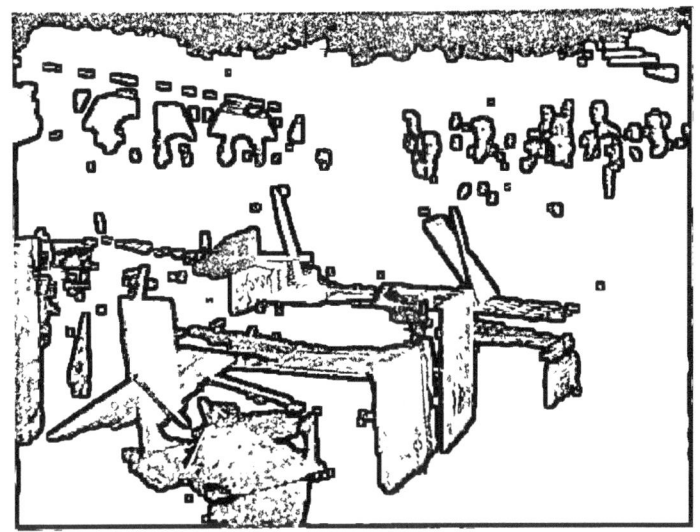

AMERICAN SANITARY TRAIN No 2
This train distributed 21 carloads of medical supplies to 217 institutions. Above,
packing cases opened for distribution at Karsk

Relief work, especially during the first year of the operation, was attended with considerable danger as the personnel were constantly exposed to every variety of infectious disease. We inoculated all Americans against cholera and the typhoid group of diseases, and vaccinated them against smallpox immediately upon arrival in Russia. They were given instructions concerning prevalent diseases, and their prevention. Large quantities of deterrents such as vermin sprays, camphor and naphthalene were kept on hand in Moscow and at district headquarters, and issued with kits of simple medicines to those about to make trips. Numerous circulars covering disease prevention were published and Supervisors and Physicians were made responsible for proper sanitation of personnel houses as well as for the observance, by personnel, of the rules laid down in our circulars. American doctors were always made available for the treatment of those contracting disease, and remained in attendance until convalescence was assured.

Inoculations and vaccinations were ordered for all Russian personnel, and we conducted dispensaries at various headquarters for these employees; that at the Moscow office alone issuing a maximum of two thousand prescriptions a month. A generous policy of granting sick leaves to those convalescing from diseases, as well as to all whose physical condition was depleted helped greatly to promote the health of our personnel.

Though we now view with considerable pride the record made by our forces in Russia, and marred by only a single death from disease the responsibility of safeguarding the health of our personnel during the trying winter of

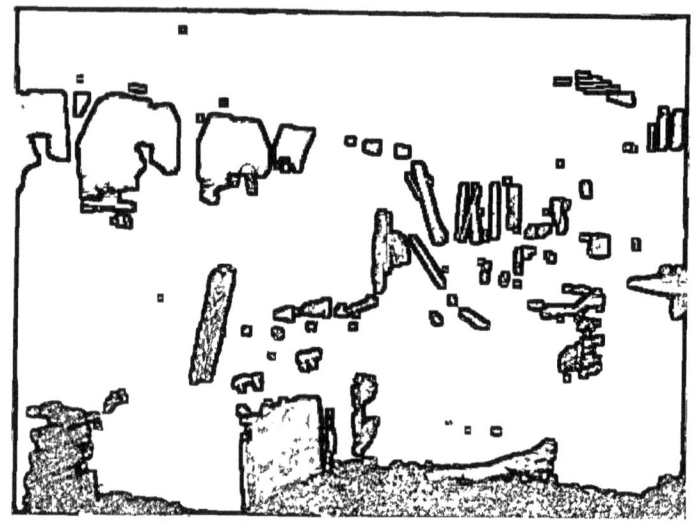

UNLOADING SUPPLIES AT TAMBOV, SANITARY TRAIN NO 2

1921 and 1922, caused us more concern than all the other difficulties which beset us.

General Medical Warehouses.

The staff consisted of from three to four Americans and a maximum of 143 Russians made up of clerks, warehousemen, watchmen, carpenters and laborers, upon American Relief Administration payrolls. In addition the government supplied seventy laborers. The administration of the warehouses and methods of handling and accounting for medical supplies will be discussed in the following chapter.

District Organization

Relief districts were territorial subdivisions of the area in which we carried out operations. These did not correspond to geographical areas as a rule, but frequently included gubernias and republics. The district of Samara was approximately the size of Virginia. Kazan, which included the Tartar Republic, Marinskaya, the Tchuvash Oblast and a portion of Perm, covered an area of over 81,000 square miles, being considerably larger than the state of Illinois. over 6,000,000 persons. Our district of Ufa, ond the border of Siberia, was roughly of the fornia, approximately 158,000 square miles. territorially, had larger populations and offered a greater opportunity for intensive work. This was especially the case in Moscow, Petrograd and the Ukraine. The latter which included four medical relief districts--Kiev, Odessa, Ekaterinoslav and Kharkov equalled Ufa in size, but had a population of over 25,000,000 persons and a correspondingly large number of medical institutions.

The local medical organizations consisted of administrative offices and medical warehouses. The personnel included the American doctors--the "District Physician"--who was in charge of the work, a second doctor or property man as assistant, during the height of the operation, and the necessary Russian personnel.

The District Physician directed all phases of the medical relief locally, but his most important duties were in connection with the supply of medical institutions. This required the development of extensive inspection and control departments to determine needs and later to check the proper use of supplies issued. Large medical warehouses were organized to receive and safeguard the supplies forwarded from Moscow and to prepare issues to institutions at hand, as well as shipments to distant points in the district.

District Physicians also initiated all measures looking toward an improvement of sanitary conditions in their areas. They conducted the various campaigns mentioned in our program, at the same time being instrumental in improving the condition of all institutions by refusing to make allocation until they had attained proper standards of cleanliness or efficiency.

Russian physicians are very high class men professionally, well educated, efficient and self-sacrificing. However, due to years of want and suffering, without facilities to combat the widespread diseases which were overwhelming the country, they had lost heart and frequently neglected the scanty resources at hand or failed to use them to great advantage. Bathing establishments and delousing apparatus, as well as much permanent equipment in hospitals, were out of commission because of the need for minor repairs. Some hospitals and many homes were filthy and badly administered because of the inertia of those in charge. Our physician being able to minister to the personal needs of the profession through the agency of food and clothing packets, and supplying them at the same time large stocks of all essentials needed by their institutions, developed great moral influence locally. They produced a marked improvement in the morale of medical personnel, which encouraged initiative and more effective use of the resources available.

The organization and administration of pharmacies and dispensaries for the treatment of general and special cases, installation of public baths, improvement of water supply, repair of hospitals and homes, the rehabilitation of laboratories, the organization of disinfecting points, and the replacing of badly administered and filthy places by model institutions were among the features included in district constructive programs. In fact, the amount of work possible in districts with good co-operation knew no limits. The organizations required to carry out this extensive program necessarily had to be large.

DEVELOPMENT OF THE PROGRAM.

The medical districts of Samara and Kazan were organized in the month of November, 1921, and a limited amount of work begun in Moscow and Petrograd. In the following month the Medical districts of Petrograd, Simbirsk, Saratov, Tzaritzin and Orenburg began operations. During the month of January, 1922, the district of Ufa was added, and by the end of this month the medical relief had been intensely developed throughout the entire Volga area.

The following telegrams from Odessa indicated the universal medical

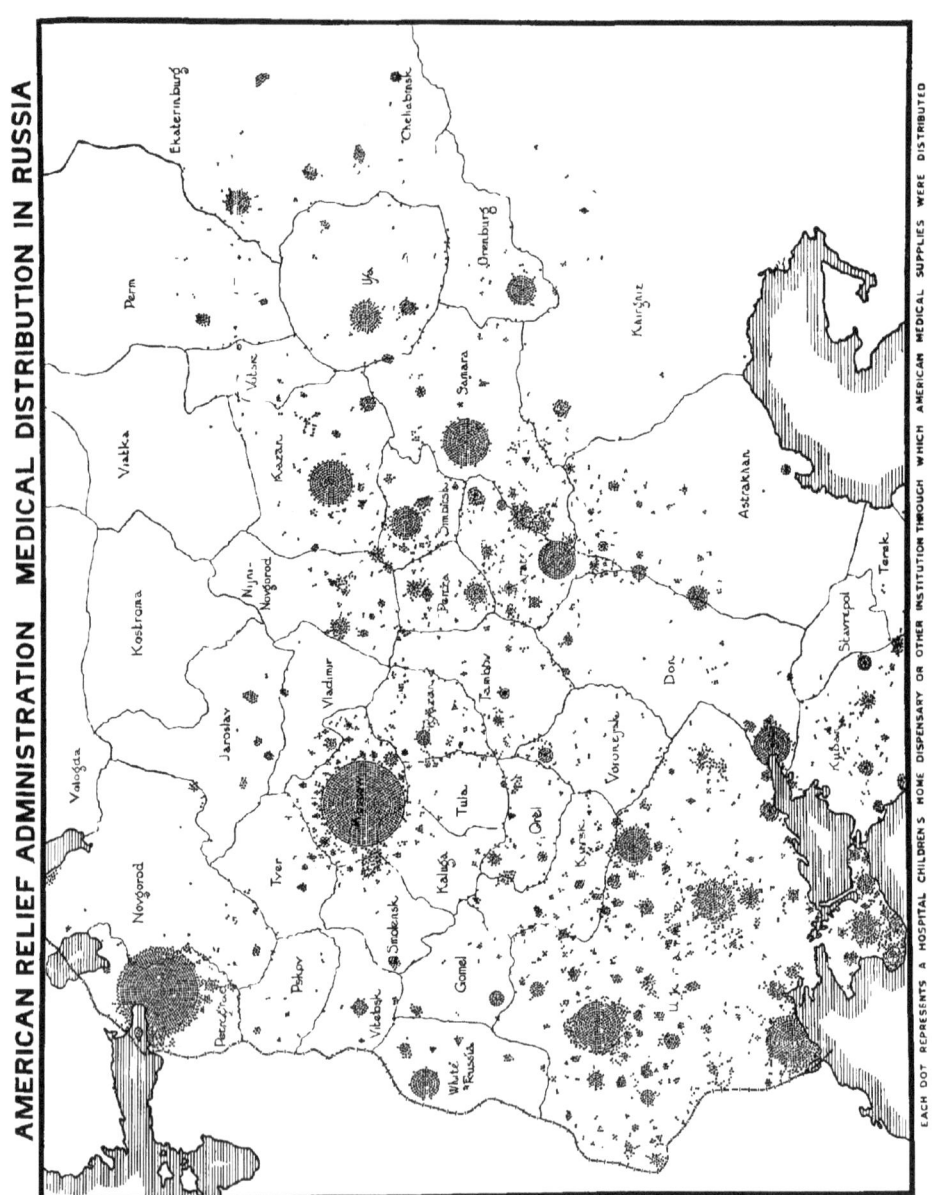

AMERICAN RELIEF ADMINISTRATION   MEDICAL DISTRIBUTION IN RUSSIA

EACH DOT REPRESENTS A HOSPITAL CHILDREN'S HOME DISPENSARY OR OTHER INSTITUTION THROUGH WHICH AMERICAN MEDICAL SUPPLIES WERE DISTRIBUTED

famine which existed:

"Over three thousand typhus and recurrent fever cases now being treated, a very difficult task due to great shortage of blankets, bedding and medicines particularly salvarsan which is most essential for treatment of recurrent fevers but practically unobtainable. Shortage blankets particularly acute. Many hospitals absolutely unheated and conditions of shivering patients, many with only one tattered blanket, is pathetic beyond words. About two hundred patients from surrounding districts arrived in Odessa daily "

"While conditions in Odessa are serious, am advised conditions in rural districts are much worse."

Conditions in South Russia, from the point of view of medical needs, did not differ materially from those existing in the Volga Basin when we began our relief operations there during the fall of 1921. This section had stood the brunt of war and revolution and numerous armies had laid it waste. Epidemics of typhus, relapsing fever and typhoid attained extreme severity in the Southern Ukraine and the cholera epidemic was more or less concentrated in this section.

At the same time medical relief in the western section of Russia became imperative, especially throughout the White Russian Republic and the gubernias of Vitebsk, Gomel, Kiev, Podolia, Volhynia and Chernigov. Most lines of communication pass across this territory and were carrying great numbers of repatriates, prisoners of war and refugees into Poland, Lithuania, and Latvia. Evacuation centers were badly administered and the hospitals and institutions caring for refugees, as well as for the local sick, were very poorly equipped. We had, therefore, by the early spring of 1922 developed sixteen separate medical relief districts covering all of Eastern, Southern and Western Russia as well as the Moscow gubernia and a considerable area to the north surrounding Petrograd. The total population of the territory in which we were operating reached approximately eighty millions.

The section left uncovered by our medical relief districts consisted of the great, sparsely populated territory in the north of Russia, as well as a wide area immediately surrounding the Moscow gubernia with numerous large cities and towns. It was entirely impractical for us to carry out relief operations in the former due to its scattered population and extremely poor transportation facilities. In the latter area, on the other hand, we operated very extensively through the agency of sanitary trains but without actually organizing relief districts.

Sanitary Train No. 1.

During the month of July, 1922, we organized Sanitary Train No. 1, consisting of twenty-one carloads of medical supplies and convoyed by Russian Red Cross Train No. 5, which was made up of dining-car, kitchen, two coaches and the supply car for soldiers of the guard. This train, in charge of Dr. Samuel B. Ross, left Moscow on August 3rd and travelled for one month. It covered approximately 2,000 miles and made distributions throughout the area, using seven of the largest cities, Tula, Orel, Kourak, Voronej, Kozlov, Tambov and Riazan as bases.

Sanitary Train No. 2.

During the months of March, April and May, 1923, we organized our Sanitary Train No. 2, in charge of Dr. John E. Toole, and distributed medical supplies through seven of the larger cities in the north, namely: Yaroslav, Kostroma, Vladimir, Ivancvo, Tver, Rybinsk and Rostov Yaroslav and to some of the smaller outlying towns. Later we covered again all of the cities in the South mentioned above and in addition, Kaluga and Bryansk. Therefore, before the close of our operation, the medical division had carried out very extensive work throughout all parts of European Russia, with the exception of the area in the northeast.

AMERICAN PERSONNEL.

Either two doctors or one doctor and one property man were assigned to practically all districts, except Tzaritzin and Orenburg, during the summer and fall of 1922. With the decision to carry on operations throughout the winter of that year our personnel was again reduced and we finally reverted to our original status of one American physician to each district. The total number of American medical personnel employed in Russia during the operation was forty-seven, made up of thirty doctors, fifteen medical property men and two stenographers, while the maximum number on duty at any one time was forty during the month of July, 1922.

The following is a list of medical relief districts with the areas covered by the same, personnel on duty in each district, as well as the approximate population of districts:

HEADQUARTERS MEDICAL DIVISION.
Moscow.

Dr. Henry Beeuwkes, Medical Director...............	Sept., 1921 to June,	1923
Dr. Walter P. Davenport, Assistant Director.........	Sept., 1921 to May,	1923
Dr. John E. Toole, Assistant......................	Nov., 1922 to June,	1923
Mr. Clyde Cleary, Assistant.......	Mar., 1922 to Sept.,	1922
Mr. Alviras Snow, Assistant................	Aug., 1922 to Sept.,	1922
Mr. J. Bentley Mulford, Assistant...................	June, 1922 to Oct.,	1922
Mr. Charles W. Surles, Assistant...................	Oct., 1922 to June,	1923
Mr. Francis P. Hogan, Secretary..	Oct., 1921 to Sept.,	1922
Mr. Arnold E. Rattray, Secretary...........	Sept., 1922 to June,	1923

Central Warehouse, Moscow.

Mr. John H. Dawson, Chief.........................	Oct., 1921 to Nov.,	1922
Mr. Rush O. Day, Assistant Chief....................	Mar., 1922 to May,	1923
Mr. Thomas J. Farraher, Assistant...................	June, 1922 to June,	1923
Mr. Charles W. Surles, Assistant...................	June, 1922 to July,	1922
Mr. Arnold E. Rattray, Secretary	May, 1922 to Sept.,	1922

Moscow District.

Territory Embraced.		Period of Service.	
Moscow City and Gubernia	Dr. W. D. Nickelsen	Mar., 1922 to Sept.,	1922
	Dr. Samuel B. Ross	Sept., 1922 to June,	1923
	Mr. John H. Raymond	June, 1922 to Oct.,	1922
4,000,000 Population	Total Russian Personnel--82		

Petrograd.

Petrograd Gubernia	Dr. Herschel C. Walker	Nov., 1921 to Oct.,	1922
Karelia Oblast	Dr. W. A. Horsely Gantt	Oct., 1922 to June,	1923
Pskov			
Tcherepovetz			
Vologda			
Novgorod			
2,500,000 Population	Total Russian Personnel--43		

Kazan District.

Tartar Republic	Mr. Stephen Venear	Oct., 1921 to Mar.,	1922

Marinski	Dr. W. R. Dear	Mar., 1922 to Nov., 1922
Chuvash	Dr. John Cox	Nov., 1922 to June, 1923
Perm ⎱ Partial	Mr. John Slack	June, 1922 to Oct., 1922
Vyatka ⎰		
6,000,000 Population	Total Russian Personnel--16	

Samara District.

Territory Embraced.		Period of Service.
Samara Gubernia	Dr. Fred H. Foucar	Jan., 1922 to June, 1923
	Dr. John E. Toole	Jan. and Feb., 1923
	Mr. Charles Hall	June, 1922 to Oct., 1922
3,500,000 Population	Total Russian Personnel--11	

Simbirsk District.

Simbirsk Gubernia	Dr. Mark L. Godfrey	Dec., 1921 to June, 1923
Penza	Mr. Ralph Z. Doty	June, 1922 to Sept., 1922
Nijni-Novgorod		
4,500,000 Population	Total Russian Personnel--21	

Ufa District.

Ufa Gubernia	Dr. Francis Rollins	Jan., 1922 to Apr., 1922
Bashkir Republic	Dr. R. McK. Sloan	Apr., 1922 to June, 1923
Tchelyabinsk	Dr. Frank R. Surber	June, 1922 to Oct., 1922
Ekaterinburg		
Kostiani		
7,812,000 Population	Total Russian Personnel--56	

Orenburg District.

Kirghiz Republic	Dr. A. B. Musa	Jan., 1922 to May, 1922
Bashkir Republic	Dr. Otto M. Beck	May, 1922 to Oct., 1922
(four cantons)		
Aktyubinsk		
2,000,000 Population	Total Russian Personnel--10	

Saratov District.

Saratov Gubernia	Dr. Jesse McElroy	Dec., 1921 to Feb., 1922
German Commune	Dr. Glenn I. Jones	Mar., 1922 to Apr., 1922
Uralsk Oblast	Dr. John E. Toole	Apr., 1922 to Nov., 1922
	Dr. W. A. Horsely Gantt	July, 1922 to Oct., 1922
	Dr. John J. Stack	Nov., 1922 to June, 1923
3,500,000 Population	Total Russian Personnel--76	

Tzaritzin District.

Tzaritzin Gubernia	Dr. George B. Cornick	Jan., 1922 to Oct., 1922
Astrakhan Gubernia	Dr. Cecil J. Handke	Oct., 1922 to Dec., 1922
	(on duty for the liquida-	
	tion of the district)	
2,000,000 Population	Total Russian Personnel--7	

Kiev District.

Kiev Gubernia	Dr. Theodore F. Foster	Mar., 1922 to May, 1923
Podolia Gubernia	Dr. Wm. E. Hurley	Nov., 1922 to Feb., 1923
Chernigov Gubernia	Mr. H. D. Brink	Aug., 1922 to Oct., 1922
Volhynia Gubernia		
9,725,000 Population	Total Russian Personnel--74	

	Odessa District.				
Kherson Gubernia	Dr. Jesse McElroy	Mar.,	1922 to May,	1922
Nikolaev Gubernia	Dr. W. R. Smith	May,	1922 to May,	1923
	Dr. E. H. Rund	July,	1922 to Oct.,	1922
6,000,000 Population	Total Russian Personnel--82			

	Kharkov District.				
Kharkov Gubernia	Dr. Frank Lyman	Mar.,	1922 to Oct.,	1922
Krementchug Gubernia	Dr. Frank Surber	Oct.,	1922 to Feb.,	1923
·	Dr. Wm. E. Hurley	Feb.,	1923 to May,	1923
	Mr. J. F. La Salle	June,	1922 to Oct.,	1923
6,665,000 Population	Total Russian Personnel--12			

	Alexandrovsk District.				
Zaporozhye Gubernia	Dr. John Caffey	June,	1922 to June,	1923
Ekaterinoslav Gubernia	Mr. Charles W. Surles	July,	1922 to Oct.,	1922
Donetz Gubernia	Mr. Renoux J. Smith	June,	1922 to Sept.,	1922
6,806,000 Population	Total Russian Personnel--16			

	Theodosia District.				
The Crimea	Mr. Stephen Venear	May,	1922 to May,	1923
1,000,000 Population	Total Russian Personnel--7			

	Rostov-Don District.				
Rostov to Trans-Caucasia	Dr. Patrick H. Kennedy	Apr.,	1922 to June,	1923
	Dr. Cecil J. Handke	June,	1922 to Feb.,	1923
	(In Tzaritzin temporarily from Oct. to Dec. of 1922)			
10,000,000 Population	Total Russian Personnel--26			

	Minsk District.				
White Russian Republic	Dr. Ralph Herz	Mar.,	1922 to Nov.,	1922
Vitebsk Gubernia	Dr. Frank Wehle	June,	1922 to May,	1923
Gomel Gubernia				
5,000,000 Population	Total Russian Personnel--18			

	Sanitary Train No. 1.	
Tula	Dr. Samuel B. Ross	Aug. and Sept., 1922
Orel		
Kursk		
Voronejh		
Riazan		
Kozlov		
Tambov	Total Russian Personnel--2	

	Sanitary Train No. 2	
Tver	Dr. John E. Toole	March
Ivanovo-Voznessensk		April } 1923
Rostov Yaroslav		May
Yaroslav		
Rybinsk		
Kostroma		
Vladimir		
Briansk		

Kaluga
And the seven other cities
mentioned above as cov-
ered by Sanitary Train
No. 1.   Total Russian Personnel--2
        The number of Russian personnel varied considerably in different dis-
tricts.

        The total maximum number of Russian employees regularly serving with
the American Relief Administration was as follows:
    Headquarters' Office and Warehouses, Moscow......................... 180
    District Organizations... 557
                                                                        ____
        Total Employees.................... 737
        In addition to the above, we temporarily employed very large numbers
of physicians, nurses and others to carry out special features of our work,
especially the inoculation program, the management of dispensaries, pharmacies, bathing institutions, et cetera. Through the generosity of Mr. William
Bingham, 2nd, of Boston, Massachusetts, we were, at all times, well supplied with
food packets, toward the close of the period with clothing packets as well, for
distribution to needy medical personnel. As many of these were only too willing to work in return for the food and clothing donated we made use of their
services in our inoculation campaign and for other special work. The maximum
number so employed at any one time reached 1,577. These were not on our pay
rolls and received no remuneration except food and clothing assistance.

CHAPTER IX

MEDICAL SUPPLIES.

PROCUREMENT.

The great bulk of American Red Cross supplies came from America, though numerous items, such as salvarsan, vaccines and antitoxins, sulphur and cod liver oil, were procured in Europe. Rapid delivery of vaccines was essential and the prices of other commodities were very much more advantageous in Europe than in America. Salvarsan, priced at seventy-five cents an ampule in America, we purchased from the French and Belgian governments at approximately ten cents a tube. As we imported 700,000 tubes into Russia during the operation, the saving on this item alone amounted to a very considerable sum of money.

Before leaving America we had arranged a "Unit Supply List," covering essential articles of the various classes of medical supplies. Unit "A" consisted of sixty-nine items of medicines, each being given a number, and the relative amounts requested made to correspond roughly with standards allowed for posts in the United States Army. Units "B," "C," "D" and "E" covered respectively, in a similar manner, disinfectants, vaccines, hospital supplies and water purification units. Requisitions by cable were prepared from time to time, requesting ten, twenty, one hundred or four hundred of these units, deleting any items, by number, not desired and doubling or trebling others required in larger amounts than specified. This system of requisitioning made for great economy and accuracy, as a cable of relatively few words could be made to cover very large quantities of medical supplies. For instance: "R. C. Requisition No...... Send one hundred units, A, B, C, fifty units D and 10 E" was interpreted as an order requesting a hundred times all of the amounts of the various drugs, disinfectants and vaccines, fifty times the amounts of hospital supplies and ten times the number of purification units covered by our unit supply tables.

As our information concerning medical needs in Russia increased, we added many additional items to our supply lists, and deleted a few of our essentials. This system of requisitioning was used until the United States Government surplus stocks began to arrive in Russia. After that period we made requisitions with a view to rounding out these supplies, and our unit supply table could no longer be used. At the same time additional resources made it possible for us to increase very considerably the variety of our stocks, so that they finally included, practically all expendable essentials needed by hospitals, laboratories and other medical institutions, and, in addition, a large amount of permanent equipment.

We had little choice in the selection of the Government Surplus stocks, for, though we had given general instructions as to the class of supplies desired in Russia, it was not possible to follow out our wishes in any detail.

Distribution.

Allocations to various districts were made primarily on a percentage basis, the following figures being given to the different districts:

Table 20

Moscow...	12%	Odessa........................	6%
Kazan....	6%	Theodosia.....................	2%
Ufa......	7%	Sanitary Train No. 1..........	2%
Petrograd..	9%	Rostov-Don....................	8%
Samara.	6%	Minsk..........	6%

Saratov....	6%	Kharkov.................	6%
Simbirsk..	6%	Ekaterinoslav.	6%
Tzaritzin.	2%	Orenburg..........	2%
Kiev.................	8%	Sanitary Train No. 2..........	2%

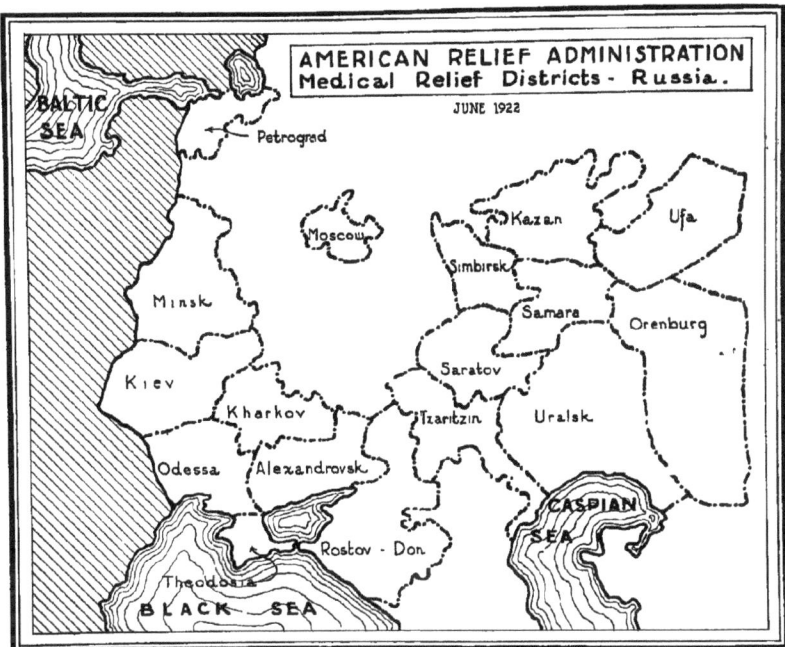

AMERICAN RELIEF ADMINISTRATION
Medical Relief Districts - Russia.
JUNE 1922

These figures were based on population of the districts, number of institutions and many other factors, and served only in a general way as a basis for allocations. They were frequently changed during the operation.

Accounting.

A satisfactory system of accounting for medical supplies, developed at the start, made proper accounting possible for all medical supplies received in Russia and the substantiation of the issues by individual receipts from each institution supplied. Red Cross supplies were covered by invoices which consisted of individual bills and packers' lists prepared by the various firms in America, from whom purchases were made. U. S. Government surplus stocks were covered by invoices prepared at the medical supply depots in America.

At the Central Warehouse, Moscow, we prepared a receiving report for the outturn of each individual car and charged ourselves upon stock record cards for all items received, identifying the supplies by case numbers on containers and corresponding invoices, or where this was impossible, by markings on cases or actual inspection of their contents. All damaged cases and those showing evidence of pilferage were opened and "Shortage--Overage Shipment Reports" prepared and appropriate entries made upon stock record cards.

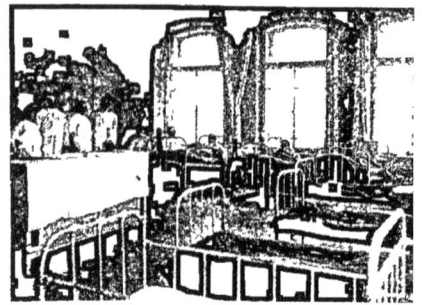

AMERICAN SURGICAL WARD EQUIPMENT IN
DR WREDEN'S HOSPITAL, PETROGRAD

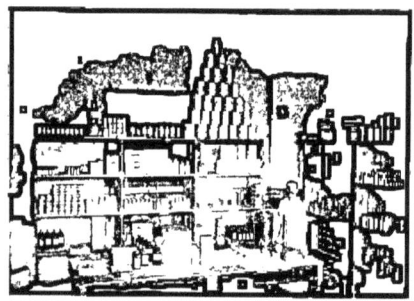

OPEN STOCK, MEDICAL WAREHOUSE, MINSK
WHITE RUSSIA

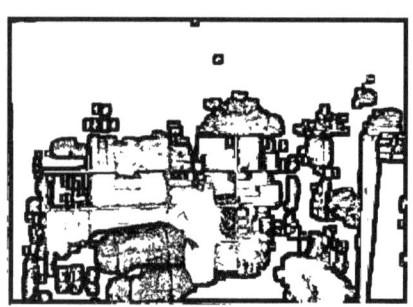

HOSPITAL SUPPLY STOCKS, MINSK, WHITE
RUSSIA, DISTRICT

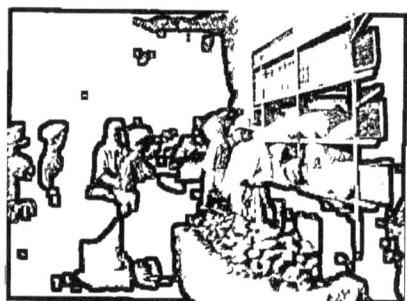

FOOD DISPENSING FOR PATIENTS IN OBOOKCOF
HOSPITAL, PETROGRAD

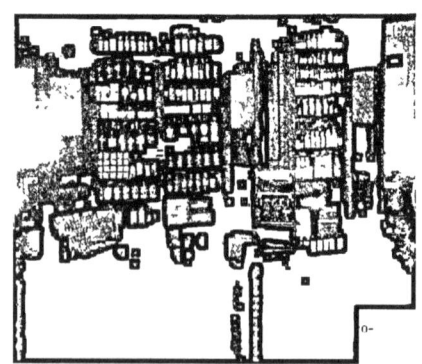

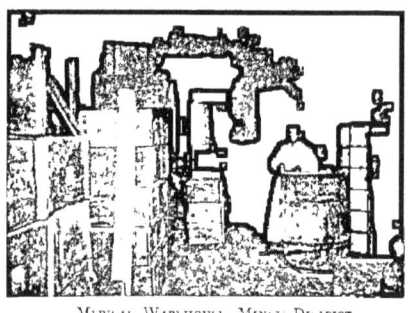

MEDICAL WAREHOUSE, MINSK DISTRICT

SCENES IN RUSSIAN HOSPITALS FURNISHED WITH AMERICAN SUPPLIES

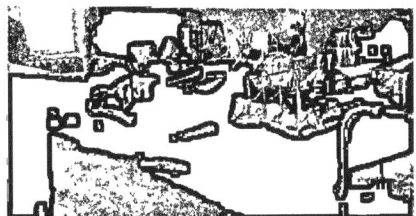

CORNER OF A CHILDREN'S WARD

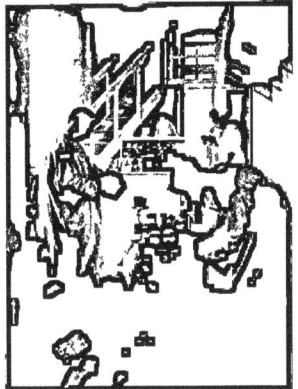

RECEIVING HOSPITAL SUPPLIES

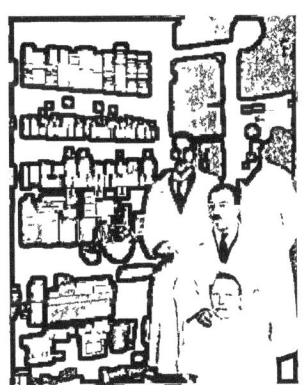

GYNECOLOGICAL CLINIC, SAMARA

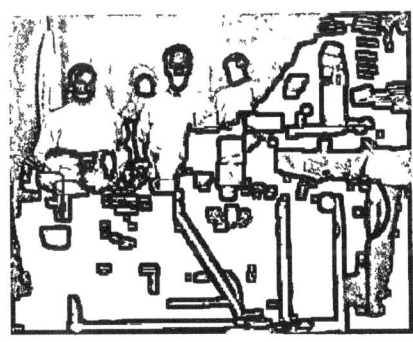

AMERICAN INSTRUMENTS FOR SAMARA
GUBERNIA HOSPITAL

AMERICAN MEDICAL SUPPLY DISTRIBUTION

Frequent inventories were made at warehouses.

All shipments to districts were made on the basis of allocations prepared at the Central Office, Moscow, and each shipment was covered by an accurate invoice and packers' list, which was forwarded by courier, while an additional packers' list was posted conspicuously with the card. Stock records were credited with all items forwarded, balances on hand being constantly current.

A commodity report was prepared monthly at the Central Warehouse, Moscow, showing amounts of each item received during the month in Moscow, as well as those shipped to each district, and balances on hand and receipts from district physicians were forwarded with these reports.

The shipments to districts were made as a rule by freight, but the courier service was used for the delivery of certain expensive supplies of small bulk, as well as in instances where the time element was important.

District physicians charged themselves upon stock record cards for all items received upon each shipment, forwarding receipts for the same to Moscow. All issues to beneficiary institutions, throughout all of our districts, were covered by accurate, detailed invoices and were signed by the personnel in charge, thus serving as receipts for the issues.

Each district prepared tri-monthly commodity reports showing in detail all supplies received from Moscow, the amounts issued to institutions, substantiated by the receipts mentioned above, as well as balances on hand. These commodity reports were checked by item at the central headquarters office at Moscow and, after necessary corrections were made, forwarded to the United States.

At the termination of the program, the Moscow office prepared a detailed consolidated commodity report covering all government surplus stocks and all Red Cross stocks handled.

The accounting for medical supplies offered many difficulties and required a tremendous amount of paper work, however, as accurate accounting induced a greater care both in distribution of supplies and their safeguarding after issue, the importance of this part of our work can hardly be overestimated.

Variety of Medical Supplies.

Medical supplies imported into Russia included 377 varieties of medicines, fifteen of disinfectants, eleven of vaccines, 133 of laboratory supplies, 627 varieties of surgical instruments, hospital and dental supplies, fifty-four of clothing and five for water purification, in all 1,222 different kinds of articles. As many of these items varied as to form, size of containers, et cetera, requiring identification on invoices, the number of items carried on stock record cards and commodity reports was much greater than 1,222. The stocks carried on government surplus were more varied than those purchased by Red Cross funds, as the former included a large number of medicines which were not absolute essentials, as well as great quantities of surgical instruments, dental supplies and hospital equipment.

Some of the supplies imported deserve special mention:

1. Hospital Bedding and Clothing.--We imported in all approximately 470,000 blankets; 570,000 bed sheets; 675,000 pairs of pajamas and night dresses, and in addition, 86,000 of layettes for infants; 890,000 towels of various kinds; 155,000 pillow cases and mattress covers and 100,000 pairs of hospital slippers. These furnished a warm bed to thousands of the sick, who

TABLE 21

Number of All Classes of Different Institutions in Russia Assisted by the Medical Division of the American Relief Administration

Cumulative to End of Each Month, November, 1921 to May, 1923

MONTHS	HOSPITALS AND SANATORIUMS		AMBULATORIES		CHILDREN'S HOMES		DAY NURSERIES		SCHOOLS		HOMES FOR AGED		OTHER INSTITUTIONS	TOTAL	
	No of Institutional	Capacity	No	Capacity	No	Capacity	No	Capacity	No	Capacity	No	Capacity	No	No	Capacity
November, 1921	28	3,778			8	1,000								36	4,778
December, 1921	306	31,180	8	296	20	4,418	1	50						335	35,944
January, 1922	567	45,605	107	1,663	79	9,132	32	1,509	8	559	19	3,482	35	847	61,950
February, 1922	1,005	58,110	275	22,564	499	21,345	40	1,970	22	1,090	35	5,891	53	1,929	111,010
March, 1922	1,362	83,749	415	45,273	743	35,239	106	2,435	29	1,525	58	9,766	78	2,791	177,987
April, 1922	2,012	110,391	630	75,840	978	53,392	161	5,810	37	2,100	73	15,341	97	3,988	262,874
May, 1922	2,328	150,418	671	84,520	1,568	89,689	203	9,650	45	3,510	73	15,341	120	5,008	353,128
June, 1922	2,760	191,520	985	95,690	1,735	108,592	224	11,385	51	3,920	95	21,297	170	6,020	432,404
July, 1922	3,199	235,703	1,681	120,823	1,974	129,832	242	15,728	69	4,899	116	34,229	240	7,521	541,214
August, 1922	4,277	246,879	2,745	170,689	2,491	178,452	256	16,660	82	5,861	146	36,464	320	10,318	655,005
September, 1922	4,353	260,180	2,970	180,604	2,761	205,093	277	17,837	94	7,063	162	41,676	390	11,007	712,453
October, 1922	4,496	274,054	3,158	191,471	3,178	223,062	324	20,358	104	7,694	169	42,439	420	11,849	759,078
November, 1922	4,542	299,010	3,338	197,783	3,344	240,098	336	20,948	120	8,614	193	50,820	510	12,383	817,273
December, 1922	4,704	310,560	3,514	207,215	3,621	255,011	348	21,098	122	9,284	205	54,253	570	13,084	857,421
January, 1923	4,869	320,909	3,632	215,537	3,768	267,621	351	21,248	125	9,881	221	58,102	630	13,596	893,298
February, 1923	5,142	325,138	3,713	224,917	4,140	297,056	354	21,464	131	10,260	222	58,143	746	14,448	936,978
March, 1923	5,298	330,037	3,680	228,111	4,345	308,798	356	21,620	139	10,316	229	58,121	814	14,861	957,003
April, 1923	5,644	346,723	3,929	243,232	4,634	329,052	368	24,109	155	12,274	245	57,048	947	15,922	1,012,938
May, 1923	5,764	353,332	4,123	247,087	4,760	336,821	372	25,259	165	17,999	248	59,237	987	16,419	1,039,735

before the winter of 1922 were being treated in unheated hospitals and with
little or no bedding except that which they supplied from their homes. Other
items in connection with ward supply included: 11,000 ice-caps; 17,000 bed-
pans; 17,000 urinals; 49,000 sputum cups; 12,000 fountain syringes; 31,000
hot water bottles and over 53,000 other items of enamel ware for ward and
operating room.

    2. Surgical Equipment.--Surgical dressings and operating room equip-
ment included, in addition to over 1,300 general and special operating sets
complete, approximately 250,000 instruments for dental and surgical use, while
dressing material in almost limitless amounts was provided, as well as
8,000,000 bandages and 86,000 bottles of collodion. These were thrown into
an absolute void. Practically nothing in the way of surgical dressings existed when we began to work.

    3. Disinfectants.--More important items among disinfectants included
2,400,000 pounds of soap; 800,000 pounds of sulphur; 200,000 pounds of cresol;
and an equal amount of formaldehyde, and over 1,000,000 pounds of chloride of
lime for the purification of water supply of cities. Over 60,000 bottles of
carbolic acid and 55,000 bottles of corrosive sublimate were also issued.

    4. Vaccines.--Vaccines included over 8,000,000 doses of tetra-vac-
cines, 4,000,000 doses of smallpox vaccines, as well as diphtheria antitoxin
and other curative sera and vaccines.

    5. Medicines.--Medicines imported in largest amounts included: Chlor-
oform and ether, forty tons; boric acid, thirty-one tons, castor oil, fifty-
seven tons; aspirin, fifteen tons; magnesia sulphate, seventy tons, and pet-
rolatum, one hundred tons. Many other drugs were imported in quantities
varying from 10,000 to 50,000 bottles.

    Probably the most popular drugs that we imported in large quantities
were quinine, neosalvarsan and cod liver oil. Its high price made quinine
practically unobtainable. Malaria was everywhere epidemic, due to absence of
this drug. We imported accordingly 60,000 pounds and distributed it widespread throughout all of our districts, inaugurating anti-malarial campaigns
in badly infected sections. We issued 700,000 tubes of neosalvarsan, its use
being limited primarily to treatment of recurrent fever, but with the great
reduction of incidence of this disease, great quantities were also used in
anti-syphilitic work. Over 700,000 pounds of cod liver oil were purchased in
Scandinavia. This made a continuous supply available to anaemic children in
all children's homes and to the general child population, through our district
dispensaries, as well as to all hospitals for the treatment of conditions incident to malnutrition. These tremendous quantities of medical supplies were
distributed broadcast to over 15,000 medical institutions administering constantly to the sick among 80,000,000 to 100,000,000 people.

RECEIPTS AND SHIPMENTS.

Number of carloads of medical supplies received in Moscow during
    the entire operation.. ....965 carloads
Number of carloads of medical supplies shipped to the various
    districts during the entire operation......................956 carloads

    The number of carloads, as well as the number of boxes, bales, bar-
rels, crates, et cetera, of medical supplies received in Moscow and shipped
to districts, by months, is as follows:

Table 22

| | Red Cross. | | | | Government Surplus. | | | |
| | Received. | | Shipped. | | Received. | | Shipped. | |
	Cars.	Cases.	Cars.	Cases	Cars.	Cases.	Cars.	Cases.
1921.								
October.. .	21	3,264	4	640	...	......	...	......
November . . .	2	358	7	1,152	...	.....	...	......
December.. ..	13	1,856	10	1,426	.	......	...	......
1922.								
January.......	8	1,111	16	2,559	...	......	..	......
February	30	3,460	23	3,422	...	......	...	......
March..	8	1,752	18	2,183	...	......	...	.....
April.... . .	56	8,994	49	7,467	..	......	...	......
May..........	43	8,C10	26	4,792	26	3,836	...	......
June...	56	6,900	40	5,571	181	31,309	106	19,797
July....	55	6,C68	65	7,572	126	21,138	86	16,277
August..... ..	82	6,604	58	4,346	44	7,550	43	7,221
September....	43	5,192	64	7,282	4	456	39	5,278
October..... ..	20	1,874	20	1,803	..	......	33	4,161
November	15	827	10	741	...	3	8	968
December.. .	20	2,530	24	2,540	..	.... .	41	6,590
1923								
January.	29	5,000	19	2,503	3	166	20	1,717
February.. ...	27	2,201	17	2,568	2	314	16	1,181
March.. . . .	21	3,478	53	8,999	...	2	6	1,656
April.	30	4,590	35	5,979	...	......	..	......
Red Cross...	579	74,069	558	73,545	386	64,774	398	64,846
Gov't Surplus	386	64,774	398	64,846	...	......	...	......
Total.....	965	138,843	956	138,391	...	......	.	......

It will be noted that the number of cars shipped was less than the number received; this is due in part to the fact that Moscow shipments were packed a little more advantageously than port shipments to Moscow, and also to small losses and breakage on route to Moscow. The discrepancies in number of containers received and shipped is due to repacking in Moscow in larger cases than those in which supplies arrived, as well as some reduction due to breakage

CHAPTER X

ASSISTANCE TO INSTITUTIONS

Assistance to all classes of medical institutions, including hospitals, ambulatories, feldsher points, disinfecting units of all varieties, laboratories of all kinds, children's homes, schools and nurseries, as well as homes for the aged and blind, was the chief function of the Medical Division of the American Relief Administration. This work was begun immediately upon our arrival in Russia and rapid and continuous progress was made up to the time the work was liquidated June 1, 1923, as demonstrated by the following tables:

Table 21 - A consolidated report showing in detail by months the total number of all classes of different institutions assisted, during the entire operation throughout all of Russia.

Table 23 - A consolidated report showing the total number of institutions assisted in each district during the entire operation.

Table 24 - A consolidated report showing the number of institutions supplied during each month.

Table 21

It will be noticed from a study of this table that thirty-six institutions, with a capacity of 4,778, were assisted in November 1921, the first month of operation, and that from this time on until September 1922 extremely rapid progress was made; that large numbers of new institutions were reached each month, and that after ten months of relief work we had assisted 10,318 institutions with a daily capacity of 655,005 patients. During July and August of 1922, tremendous amounts of surplus government medical stocks arrived in all districts, including numerous items not previously issued. These were now allocated to the institutions previously assisted. At the same time our district physicians continued to reach institutions not previously covered because they were in more isolated areas out of touch with transport. The great majority of accessible institutions in older districts had been reached by September 1922, and many had received frequent issues covering all classes of supplies. Our report shows accordingly a more gradual increase in the number of new institutions reached monthly after this time. Many of these were in areas outside of original district borders and later included as we increased the size of our districts. During the first year of operations we had reached 13,084 medical institutions with a capacity of 857,421, and during the entire program of approximately nineteen months' work, we assisted 16,419 institutions of all classes with a daily total capacity of 1,039,735.

It will be noted that 987 "other institutions," not included under hospitals, homes, et cetera, received aid from the Medical Division of the American Relief Administration. These included laboratories, disinfecting points, and camions, inoculation companies, water purification units, et cetera. Their capacity is not stated, as obviously they were not concerned in the treatment of the sick, and in this sense had no capacity. However, the influence of our aid in assisting these institutions organized for the prevention of disease can be scarcely over-estimated.

Table 23

This table, showing the number of all classes of different institutions assisted in each district during the whole operation, demonstrated the wide distribution of medical stocks throughout practically all of European Russia.

-97-

TABLE 23

Number of Institutions in Russia assisted by The American Relief Administration

November, 1921—June, 1923

DISTRICTS	HOSPITALS AND SANATORIUMS		AMBULATORIES		CHILDREN'S HOMES		DAY NURSERIES		SCHOOLS		HOMES FOR AGED		OTHER INSTITUTIONS	TOTAL	
	No of Institutions	Capacity	No.	Capacity	No.	Capacity	No.	Capacity	No.	Capacity	No.	Capacity	No.	No of Institutions	Capacity
Moscow	539	47,441	130	40,264	755	53,990	167	9,256	12	657	13	2,294	154	1,770	153,902
Petrograd	521	34,573	333	50,669	487	20,844	10	791	20	6,192	63	19,071	139	1,573	132,140
Kazan	323	17,020	192	3,721	91	8,373	36	3,364	14	501	2	30	36	694	33,009
Simbirsk	276	18,011	316	11,220	321	25,201	42	2,628	38	2,984	18	1,606	5	1,016	61,650
Samara	163	8,124	168	10,644	159	12,576	.		14	1,213	6	403	70	580	32,960
Ufa	372	23,951	229	1,196	355	32,341	4	206	29	2,305	2	260	28	1,019	60,259
Orenburg	87	6,144	142	5,962	86	9,144			3	420	15	3,513	4	337	25,183
Saratov	358	19,240	488	10,677	488	34,119	49	5,099	7	309	55	13,648	69	1,514	83,092
Tzaritzin	143	8,276	83	3,303	40	4,833					5	13,422	19	290	29,834
Rostov	340	22,946	152	11,504	341	27,221			1	200	3	60	90	927	61,931
Kharkov	509	26,744	247	13,066	84	6,919					5	646	38	883	47,375
Kiev	489	27,015	281	13,949	731	37,036	15	614	2	41	10	753	49	1,577	79,408
Odessa	246	16,776	126	5,473	239	16,644	12	617	6	1,194	12	1,126	69	710	41,830
Minsk	220	18,979	155	13,297	100	6,580	8	258	9	1,165	20	1,686	75	587	41,965
Crimea	111	5,355	171	4,852	193	17,299	13	906	9	768	10	464	68	575	30,144
Ekaterinslav	402	20,348	252	22,458	239	19,877	11	1,306	.		6	135	71	981	64,124
Sanitary Train No 1	502	21,565	639	20,803	21	1,727	3	125	1	50	3	120		1,169	44,390
Sanitary Train No 2	163	10,824	19	4,029	30	1,597	2	89					3	217	16,539
Total	5,764	353,332	4,123	247,087	4,760	336,821	372	25,259	165	17,999	248	59,237	987	16,419	1,039,735

Table 24

This table shows the number of institutions supplied each month. The total number of different issues of medical supplies reached something over 40,000, which made an average of slightly under three issues to each institution assisted. The number of issues to hospitals, ambulatories, homes, et cetera, varied very considerably. Some of those in the cities where headquarters were located were supplied at frequent intervals and given relatively smaller amounts of the expendable articles in order to conserve our stocks and retain a maximum of control. On the other hand, institutions at great distances from our bases of supplies, and especially those located in isolated sections, received larger issues at greater intervals, and some of these received in all only one initial and one final issue. Again, hospitals and homes assisted by our Sanitary Train No. 1 received one issue in August of 1922, and the more important and accessible ones were again covered in the spring of 1923. Those supplied north of Moscow gubernia received only one issue from Sanitary Train No. 2. The hospitals and homes, on the other hand, assisted through our regular district organizations, received an average of over three issues.

NATURE OF ASSISTANCE.

Hospitals.--In making distributions, especially of non-expendable articles, the effectiveness of the administration of hospitals received special consideration, and issues to those well administered naturally surpassed those institutions of a lower standard.

Bedding and Ward Equipment.--Our allowance of bedding for the average well-managed hospital totaled a maximum of two blankets, four sheets, two to four towels and two to four pairs of pajamas and night dresses per bed. Bed pans and urinals were distributed roughly on a basis of one for ten beds with a proportionate allowance of hot water bottles and ice bags, thermometers, syringes, and rectal tubes, et cetera. In making issues, district physicians of course took into consideration the equipment on hand, and made their allocations with a view to bringing up the bedding and ward equipment supply to the standard we aimed to reach. The many institutions of a temporary character, and those with great numbers of temporary beds during the epidemic periods, we could not bring up to standards mentioned above though we gave them supplies sufficient to assist them during the emergency. Even toward the close of our operation we were still supplying new institutions. All district physicians reported their permanent hospitals, at the close of the period, in a very satisfactory condition as regards bedding and equipment.

Surgical Needs.--Our supplies of general surgical instruments, which included 648 general operating cases, 367 cases of hemostatic forceps, 435 smaller cases of instruments, and 572 medical and surgical chests as well as approximately 250,000 surgical and dental instruments, helped to fill a great need in rounding out instrumentariums on hand. They made possible the rehabilitation of very many surgical clinics. Our surgical sets for specialties including 336 genito-urinary cases, 156 ear, nose and throat cases, and 136 eye cases were sufficient to place practically all the special departments of hospitals in a satisfactory situation as regards surgical instruments. The supply of smaller hospitals with surgical equipment was of special importance. These institutions were practically without instruments and many had previously been unable to handle satisfactorily even their minor surgical cases.

When we began work Russia had almost no surgical dressings and bandages. Our tremendous issues made possible a great increase in the number of operations, the proper treatment of wounds, as well as marked improvement in surgical technique and reduction in infections. District Physicians reported

-99-

the supply of surgical dressings on hand in hospitals as sufficient to permit of continued operation for from three to six months after the termination of our program.

Large varieties of enamel ware, including basins, pans, pails, trays, cups, et cetera, in United States Government stocks, received the wildest distribution, as did the numerous operating tables of all types, made for great improvement in the appearance of hospitals, dispensaries and homes and brought great comfort to the sick. Mess chests and chests of cooking utensils, as well as large cups, etc., in U. S. Government stocks, received the wildest distribution, as quantities of separate dishes, pots, pans and table-ware were important items, for hospitals and institutions had frequently only wooden spoons and bowls in such insufficient quantity that only a few of the inmates or patients could be fed at one time. Great numbers of oil stoves, lamps, commode chests, et cetera, were issued. Such semi-permanent equipment had long ago worn out or been lost and replacement by poverty-stricken institutions had been impossible. Such permanent apparatus as Albee Bone sets, Hudson trephines, cystoscopes, electric ophthalmoscopes, et cetera were also received in relatively large numbers. Though not absolute essentials, they greatly complemented hospital equipment. Though no relief organization could cover the needs for permanent equipment in hospitals and homes in Russia, our large issues did serve to materially improve the appearance of institutions. They made possible much more effective treatment of the sick and care of children in homes. They raised the morale of medical personnel.

Radiographic tubes and plates, issued toward the close of our operation, filled a great want, as many hospitals had good general X-ray equipment, but were unable to carry out any work due to the fact that their supply of tubes had become exhausted. Because these tubes were very expensive, they were highly treasured by the few institutions that received them. They made possible continued operation for a long period of numerous radiographic laboratories which would have closed had it not been for our aid.

Medicines and Expendable Supplies.--American medicines and other expendable articles covered the needs of hospitals for practically all essentials during the entire period of our operations. At the termination of our program, institutions were issued sufficient supplies to care for their needs during a period of from three to six months, and have many items in sufficient quantities to carry them on for a year.

Children's Homes.

Issues to children's homes, as well as to hospitals varied with the effectiveness and efficiency of their administration. Often we were able to turn filthy and badly organized children's homes into well administered institutions by the encouragement of supplying them with the means to attain cleanliness and order. Issues to homes included large numbers of blankets, sheets, children's clothing and quantities of heavy wool underwear. Drugs of the simpler sort were issued to homes, making treatment of minor illnesses possible, especially that of ever present skin diseases and eye affections. Some surgical instruments, and dressings, iodine and disinfectants were distributed as well, while all larger homes, having infirmary beds for their sick, were supplied with the essentials generally issued to smaller hospitals.

Soap, sulphur, cresol and formaldehyde were freely issued. They were a great factor in improving sanitary conditions and eliminating infectious diseases.

TABLE 24

Number of Institutions in Russia Supplied Each Month by the American Relief Administration

MONTHS	HOSPITALS AND SANATORIUMS No of Institutions	Capacity	AMBULATORIES No	Capacity	CHILDREN'S HOMES No	Capacity	DAY NURSERIES No	Capacity	SCHOOLS No	Capacity	HOMES FOR AGED No	Capacity	OTHER INSTITUTIONS No	TOTAL No of Institutions	Capacity
November, 1921	28	3,778			8	1,000								36	4,778
December, 1921	306	31,180	8	296	20	4,418	1	50						335	35,944
January, 1922	272	19,231	157	8,717	143	21,203	12	870			10	2,100	6	600	52,121
February, 1922	450	41,965	91	7,260	297	31,535	22	1,310	3	140	7	1,558	13	883	83,868
March, 1922	488	41,168	317	12,413	252	21,300	62	3,454	6	450	13	1,381	18	1,156	80,156
April, 1922	561	69,791	222	23,385	291	36,077	16	1,048	8	770	34	2,100	16	1,148	133,171
May, 1922	800	93,275	362	48,522	620	34,359	50	2,500	8	602	27	4,411	39	1,904	183,669
June, 1922	1,093	94,446	508	55,557	613	45,592	120	8,488	6	2,061	41	5,035	55	2,466	211,179
July, 1922	1,663	120,858	818	73,329	662	49,457	86	4,775	36	3,196	25	2,605	55	3,470	254,220
August, 1922	1,837	137,149	1,477	93,627	892	75,698	31	1,927	46	2,074	55	7,601	170	4,787	318,076
September, 1922	782	48,622	548	33,655	651	55,122	44	4,711	38	2,949	24	1,929	155	2,342	146,988
October, 1922	973	82,677	527	40,817	1,308	77,953	77	4,143	29	2,240	24	4,766	83	3,021	212,596
November, 1922	928	103,512	475	50,707	534	50,318	33	2,092	35	2,955	18	8,261	118	2,141	217,845
December, 1922	759	59,288	448	45,293	985	108,550	55	2,953	26	3,486	33	7,162	98	2,404	227,272
January, 1923	751	67,204	638	51,024	574	50,950	59	3,649	32	4,498	32	4,985	77	2,163	182,310
February, 1923	918	78,697	810	63,629	767	77,649	77	4,621	59	8,214	17	1,916	141	2,789	234,726
March, 1923	948	60,190	995	52,737	881	83,189	54	3,007	34	3,668	22	2,838	170	3,104	205,629
April, 1923	1,628	122,760	973	203,351	1,026	90,097	21	742	62	7,512	52	6,007	410	4,172	430,469
May, 1923	799	88,183	405	147,253	472	50,536	3	170	22	7,343	5	3,305	166	1,872	296,790

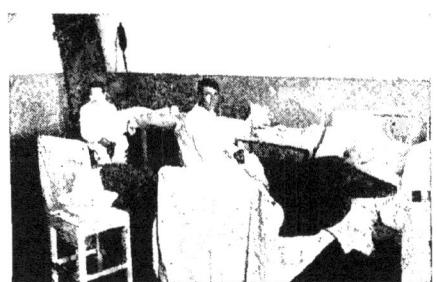

MEN'S WARD OF A GOVERNMENT HOSPITAL

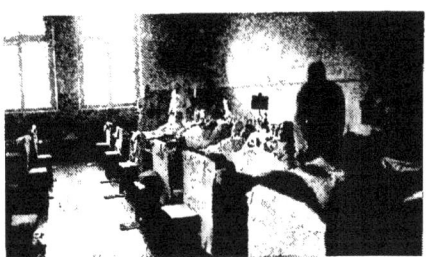

A CITY HOSPITAL

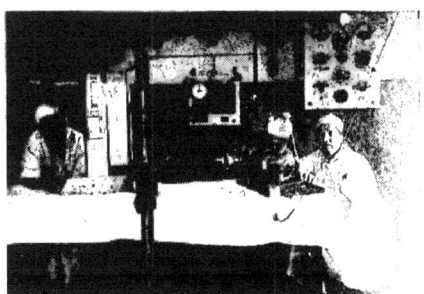

RADIOGRAPHIC EQUIPMENT

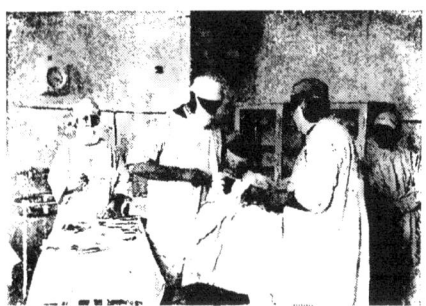

A SURGICAL CLINIC

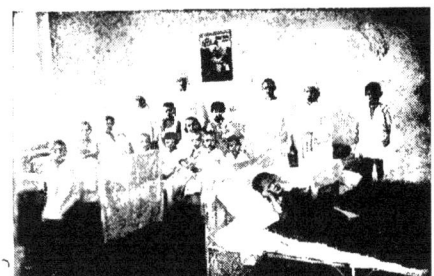

CHILDREN'S WARD IN A THERAPEUTIC
HOSPITAL

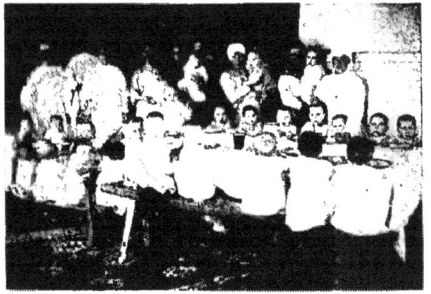

DINING ROOM IN A CHILDREN'S HOME

VIEWS IN RUSSIAN INSTITUTIONS
All American Equipment and Supplies

Cod liver oil was distributed broadcast to all homes and reports from district physicians indicate that its universal use had great influence in improving the physical condition of the children and influencing favorably the various deficiency diseases, which were so common

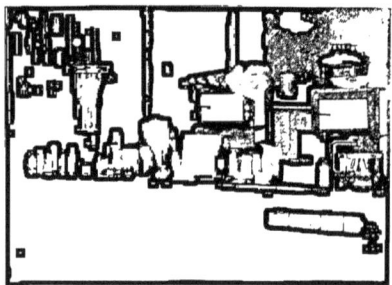 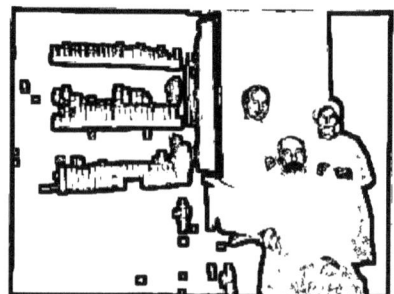

THE ROUX LABORATORY, SAMARA RUSSIA
An illustration of the varied nature of the medical assistance rendered Russian institutions
This laboratory was supplied with drugs and equipment so its important work could be carried on

Assistance to Ambulatories.

This was just as important as aid to hospitals, for dispensaries had become entirely devoid of supplies and could give patients nothing more than advice and prescriptions. They had no medicines to issue and could make not even emergency dressings. Our issues included all classes of medicines and large amounts of surgical dressings, as well as considerable quantities of permanent equipment. Soap, vaccines and disinfectants were issued through these dispensaries in large amounts, as well as huge quantities of badly needed cod liver oil.

Laboratories.

The importance of our aid to laboratories can scarcely be overestimated The Roux Laboratory at Samara was completely supplied by a special purchase made in America and was continuously assisted throughout the operation. Through American aid it was converted from a paralyzed and demoralized organization, producing nothing, into a most active and effective institution manufacturing all varieties of vaccines and sera in quantity, and carrying out important bacteriological and analytical work for surrounding hospitals.

Laboratory supplies consisted of all varieties of stains reagents, glassware, culture media, and limited amounts of the various sugars needed in bacteriological diagnosis Large numbers of haemocytometers, haemoglobinometers, and urinometers were also provided, as well as autoclaves, sterilizers, and other permanent equipment in considerable amounts. We distributed about a hundred and fifty microscopes among high class laboratories, and a limited number to a few of the well established medical universities Issues to laboratories made possible not only a great improvement in diagnostic medicine preparation of sera and vaccines so important in

d blind were assisted similarly to children's homes.

<u>American Relief Administration Dispensaries and Pharmacies.</u>

A considerable number of American Relief Administration dispensaries and pharmacies were also organized. Under the New Economic Policy many institutions made charges for medicines and there was a tendency to give preference to certain classes to the exclusion of others. Our dispensaries and pharmacies, organized where ambulatory facilities were lacking or insufficient, served a wonderful purpose in providing effective medical attention for tremendous numbers of sick. They brought relief directly to thousands.

<u>Moscow Central Dispensary</u> --This institution comprised fifteen departments: Therapeutic, Pediatric, Surgical, Nervous, Gynecological, Venereal, Urological, Ear, Nose and Throat, Eye, Dental, Psychiatrical, Laboratory and Pharmacy The daily capacity was about five hundred prescriptions and the various departments could handle upwards of three hundred patients daily. Children's homes were supplied from this dispensary About 1,200 prescriptions for students were filled monthly. The remainder of the patients were American Relief Administration Russian employees, the unemployed and invalids. The Dental Department had four dentists who handled about fifteen patients daily. The highest number of prescriptions filled in a single month was 14,000. This organization was turned over to the Bureau of Unemployment, who will continue to operate it for the unemployed.

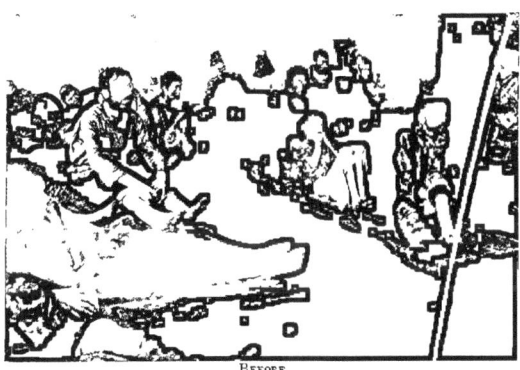
BEFORE

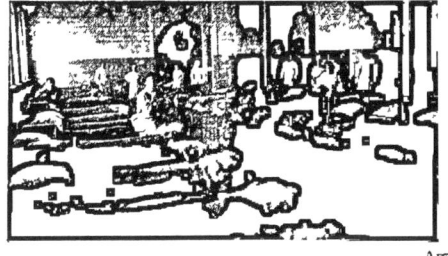 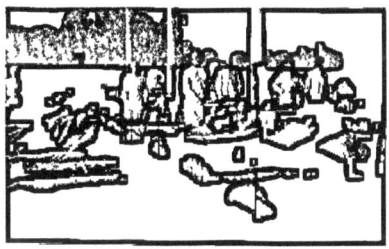
AFTER

HOSPITAL NO 920, CHELIABINSK
A sample of how thousands of hospitals looked before arrival of American aid in the famine
of 1921, and after supplies arrived

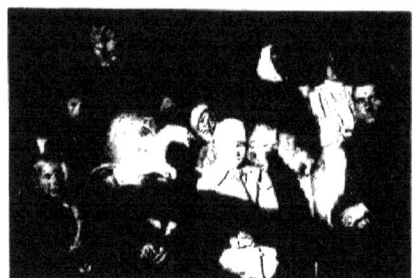

RAILROAD STATION DISPENSARY WAITING ROOM

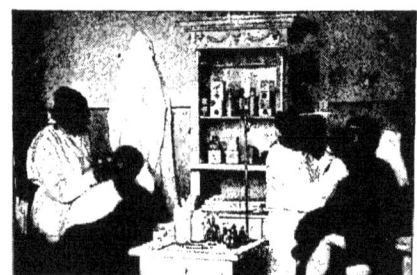

DENTAL AMBULATORY

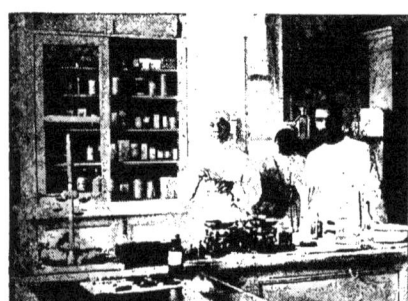

DISPENSARY SUPPLY SECTION

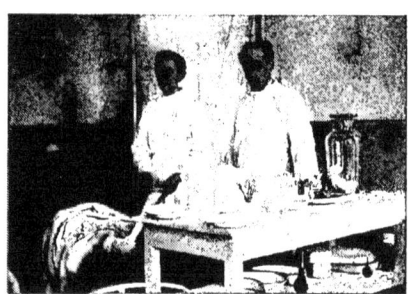

CITY DISPENSARY

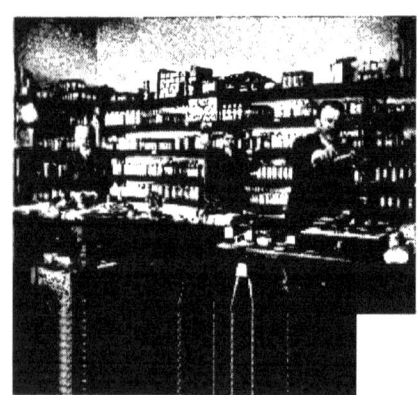

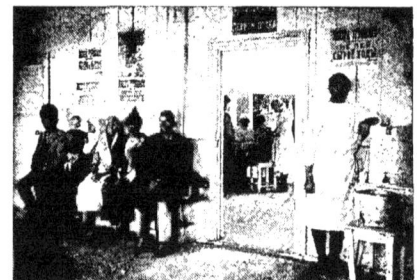

REFUGEE DISPENSARY

MEDICAL AID IN THE RUSSIAN FAMINE
A few of the varied institutions assisted

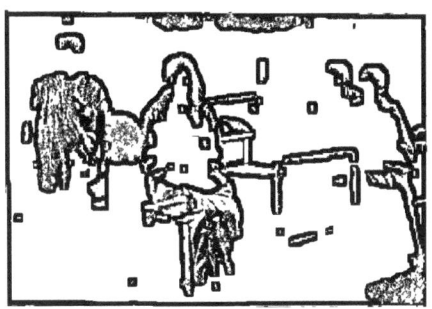

WOMEN'S WARD

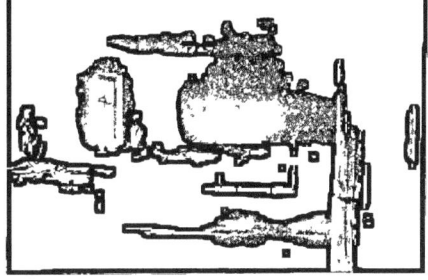

ISOLATION WARD

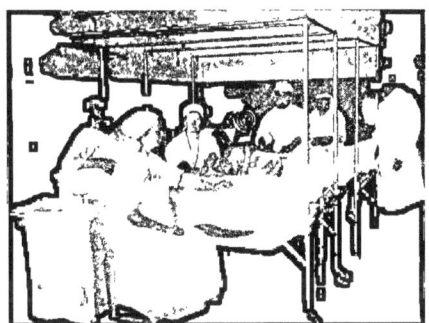

SURGICAL WARD WITH FRACTURE BEDS

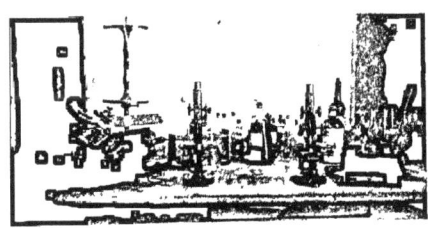

LABORATORY SUPPLIES AND EQUIPMENT

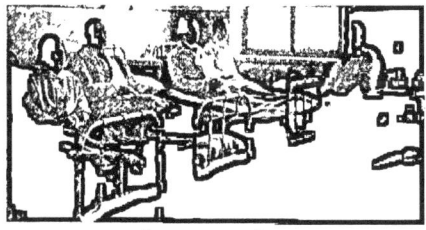

GYNECOLOGICAL CLINIC

RUSSIAN HOSPITAL SCENES
With American Equipment

The American Relief Administration Headquarters Dispensary treated a maximum of 1,000 patients a month mainly, but not exclusively, employees of the American Relief Administration.

Kiev City.--The first dispensary was organized in Kiev City in May, 1922, treating twenty patients the first day and between 140 and 170 daily after the first few weeks. It made 300 inoculations per day during the American inoculation campaign. The need for medical relief of this kind was so great in Kiev, that Dr. Foster established three other dispensaries in different parts of the city. During the latter months each of the four averaged 170 treatments daily. A Roentgen cabinet for radiographic diagnosis, a laboratory for analysis and a dental dispensary were also established, the latter being one of the finest and best equipped in the city of Kiev, and the first free dental dispensary organized in that town. The number of patients treated in these dispensaries totalled 121 271 and the number of prescriptions issued 107,032. A dispensary was also organized at Vinnitsa treating daily from forty to fifty patients. This organization was turned over to the Joint Distribution Committee at the close of our program to continue its operation.

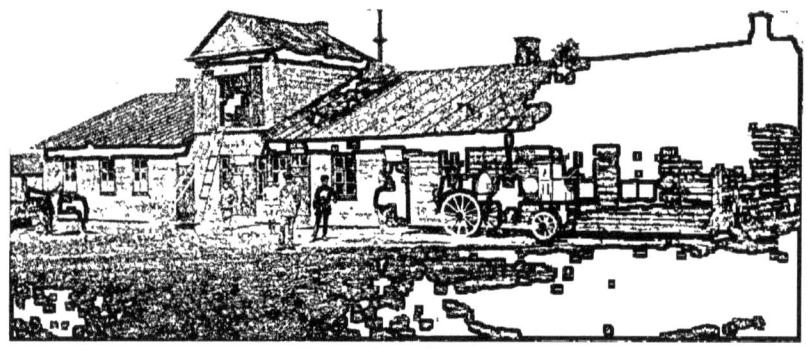

RUSSIAN PUBLIC BATH HOUSE
With one of the French Disinfectors supplied by the A R A in its war on typhus lice

Simbirsk.--The American Relief Administration established twenty-two dispensaries, pharmacies and other organizations in the Simbirsk district, treating or providing medicines for an average of 2,574 patients daily. Most of these were for the treatment of general cases, but a large malaria station was organized at Penza and is at present treating 250 malaria cases each day. Dr. Godfrey also organized a laboratory at Rozaevka for railroad hospitals of the Moscow-Kazan Railroad. This was the only institution of its kind within a wide radius. Another laboratory was organized in Simbirsk city, at the Children's Hospital, to take care of this institution and the various local children's homes. Most of these organizations will continue to operate as they were well supplied at the termination of our program.

well supplied at the the the A.R.A. dispensary treated a maximum of 400
well supplied at the the dicines to between 300 to 400. In addition a
well supplied at the the for 250 needy each day and three Baby Consulta-
well supplied at the the aximum of 575 babies and filled 300 prescriptions
a day.

Ufa.--A large pharmacy was organized in the city of Ufa to care for patients, who passed through city ambulatories but were unable to secure medi-

-107-

cines, as well as to provide for the needs of all children's homes. A similar pharmacy was established at Sterlitamak and these two organizations provided medicines for a maximum of 250 patients daily. Ambulatories were also organized in Ufa and Ekaterinburg, treating a maximum of 250 patients each day.

Rostov-Don.--The American Relief Administration pharmacy at Novotcharkask provided medicines for 300 patients a day. Two malaria stations established at Rostov, treated over 300 malaria cases daily. A pharmacy was also organized at Rostov to take care of the needs of eighty-five children's homes there.

Petrograd.--In addition to supplying 265 dispensaries in the city of Petrograd, the A.R.A. set up an ambulatory at the main office with a dental cabinet. Four dispensaries at Student Kitchens, and two in children's kitchens were established, treating 175 patients a day as well as filling 250 prescriptions. First Aid stations were provided as well, in all of the kitchens in which we fed.

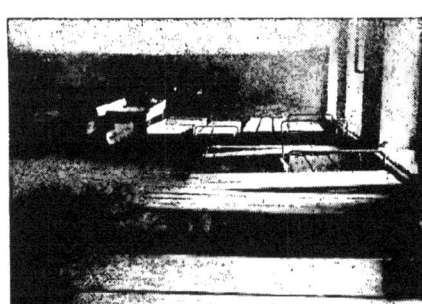

BEFORE SUPPLIES ARRIVED   AFTER

RECEIVING HOME FOR WAIFS, SARATOV

Crimea.--Here the A.R.A. established three dispensaries, treating 100 patients daily.

Ekaterinoslav.--A very large A.R.A. at Ekaterinoslav city treated over 400 patients daily, and provided approximately 200 home visits a month. A pharmacy, working in conjunction with this dispensary provided medicines for 250 persons daily.

Odessa.--Four dispensaries and one pharmacy were organized, treating over 400 patients daily and issuing prescriptions to 500.

Kazan.--Three ambulatories treating 325 patients daily were organized; also a trachoma institute with a bed capacity of seventy devoted exclusively to treatment of trachoma cases. This was probably the only institution of its kind in Russia.

Orenburg.--One large ambulatory and a separate pharmacy were founded by the American Relief Administration. The former treated eighty to ninety patients daily and the pharmacy filled approximately 300 prescriptions per day.

Samara.--Probably no dispensaries organized by the American Relief Administration were of more importance from the point of view of disease pre-

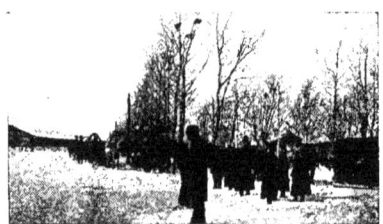

MEDICAL SUPPLIES IN TRANSIT TO HOSPITALS
IN PENZA

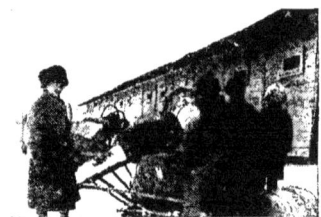

TO OUTLYING DISTRICTS IN NIJNI
NOVGOROD

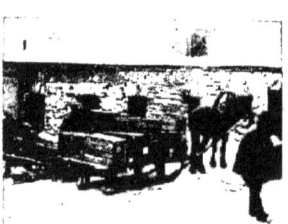

TYPICAL RUSSIAN SLEDGES
WITH MEDICAL SUPPLIES

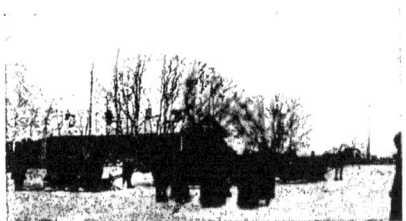

OFF TO COUNTRY REGIONS IN SIMBIRSK

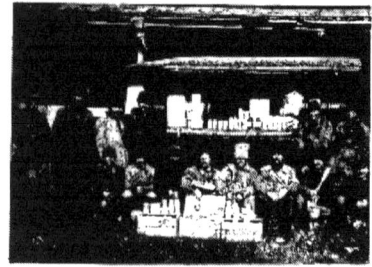

A R A MEDICAL AUTOMOBILE SAMARA

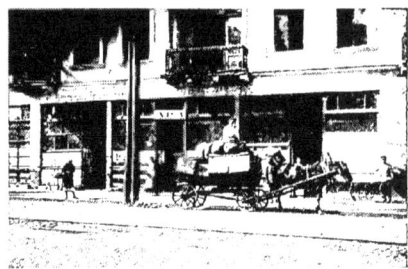

THE START OF AN AWKWARD TRIP TO MINSK
COUNTRY HOSPITALS

SUPPLIES TO COUNTRY DISTRICTS

After all the troubles of shipping supplies overseas and pushing them through over Russia's broken-down railways, the long hauls over impassable Russian roads were often the most difficult stages of the journey

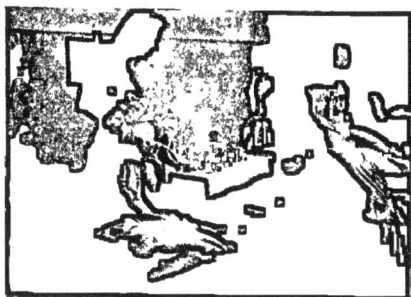

ADMINISTERING NEOSALVARSAN

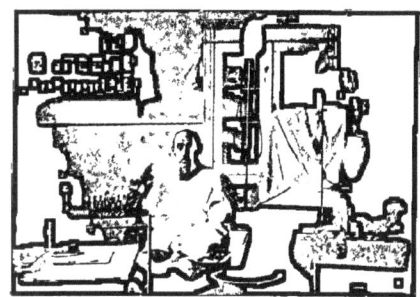

SYPHILITIC SECTION, SAMARA VENEREAL DIS-
PENSARY

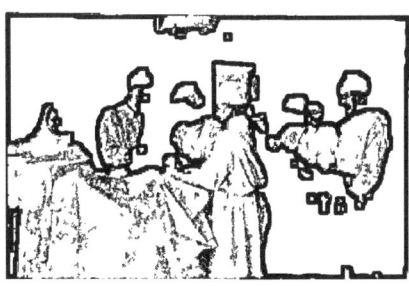

AMERICAN SURGICAL SUPPLIES IN OPERATING
ROOMS

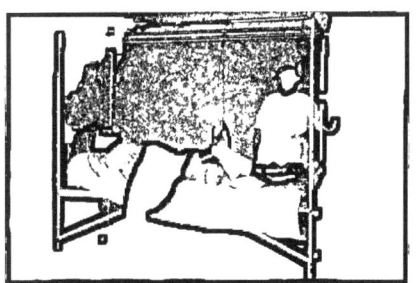

FRACTURE BED

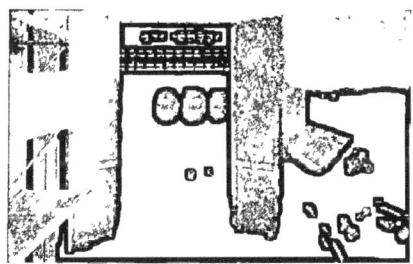

HOSPITAL FOOD RATIONS

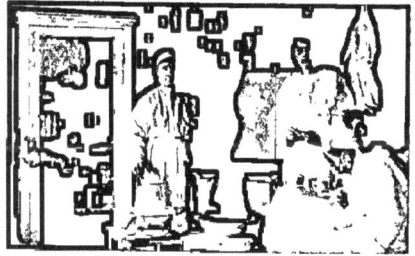

SKIN TREATMENT DISPENSARY

RUSSIAN HOSPITALS

The above series of photographs show the well-rounded nature of the American assistance to over 5,000 Russian
hospitals, all supplies o equipment furnished by the A R A

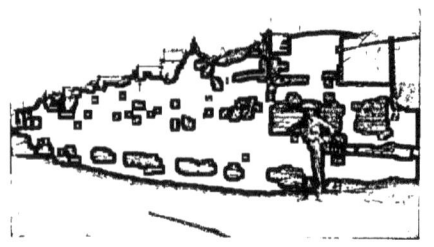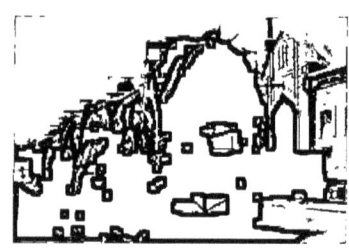

THE COMBAT OF TYPHUS
Disinfectors for lice elimination ready to be rushed to refugee camps in famine areas

vention than those established at the railroad stations, in the Samara district. Samara is the main junction point for railroads passing from Turkestan and Siberia into European Russia and one of the most important portals of entry of disease.

1. A.R.A. Ambulatory, Samara City Railroad Station.

This dispensary was organized October 5th, 1922, for the examination and treatment of all refugees passing through Samara city by train, and for the prompt isolation of those suffering from infectious diseases.

Table 25

Number of trains inspected in this dispensary	868
Patients removed from trains to dispensary	1,030
Patients removed from station to dispensary	2,427
Patients removed from dispensary to hospital	2,339
Dead bodies removed from trains and railroad stations	26
Total patients attended to	12,077
Prescriptions filled	75,000

Patients suffering from infectious diseases and removed from trains and isolated were as follows:

Typhus Exanthematicus	48
Typhus Recurrentis	231
Typhus, undiagnosed type	634
Malaria	1,231
Scarlet Fever	3
Influenza	658
Diphtheria	1
Measles	24
Smallpox	3
Scurvy	20
Dysentery	106
Mumps	7
Erysipelas	11
Syphilis	132
	127
	8
ases	238

-111-

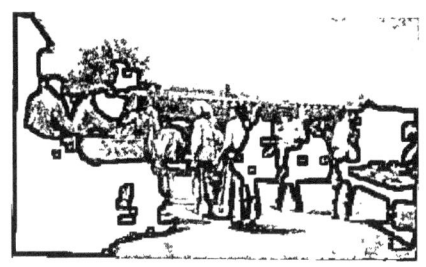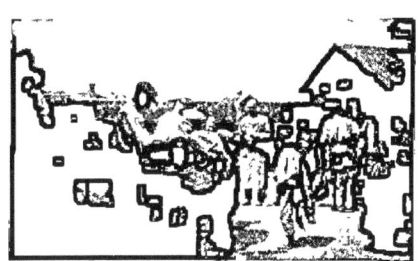

PEASANT REFUGEES RECEIVING TYPHOID-CHOLERA INOCULATION AT EMERGENCY STATION

There were in addition 2,583 minor surgical cases and 5,912 unclassified.

2. A R A. Dispensary, Kinel R. R. Station.

This dispensary was established to act as a check upon the influx of contagious diseases by refugee trains from Siberia.

Total number of patients treated in this dispensary . . .   5,456
Number of trains inspected...   102
Sick removed from trains to dispensary   441
Dead bodies removed from trains   21

The type of disease treated and isolated corresponded closely to those mentioned above for the Samara dispensary.

The importance of early detection and isolation of these refugees suffering from infectious diseases in preventing the spread of infectious diseases cannot be over estimated.

3. A.R.A. Dispensary at Stavropol treated 1,500 patients monthly.

4. A R.A. Dispensary, Arezni Dom, Samara City treated 1,500 patients per month.

5. A R.A. Dispensary, Samara City. This institution was designed mainly to care for A R.A. employees on duty and 4,814 were treated all told.

6. A.R.A. Free Bath Dispensary. This dispensary was established to give free medical aid to the population receiving free bathing facilities. The number of patients treated during its operation was 4,495.

Aid to Medical Personnel.

The generosity of Mr. William Bingham, 2nd, of Boston, who donated $95,000 for food and clothing packets for the medical personnel of Russia enabled the A.R.A. throughout the entire program to render very material and continued relief to doctors, nurses and attendants.

The actual distribution of these packets was made by our district's physicians to whom we allocated as follows:

Table 26

District.	No. of Food Packets	No. of Clothing Packets
Moscow..	409	80
Petrograd..	400	80
Kazan.......	782	100
Forwarded..	1591	260

Brought forward.	1591	260
Minsk.........	400	100
Rostov-Don....	475	100
Saratov.	515	100
Kiev...	500	75
Odessa........ . . .	558	80
Ekaterinoslav.	275	75
Simbirsk.	475	100
Ufa....	525	100
Orenburg...	200	...
Samara	845	120
Kharkov	175	75
Simferopol	225	50
Tzaritzin.....	125	.
Individual allocations by Dr. Beeuwkes to physicians in Moscow	16	15
	6,900	1,250

The food and clothing packets donated by Dr. Henry O. Eversole were distributed through the District Physicians of the American Relief Administration as follows:

Table 27

District.	No. of Food Packets.	No of Clothing Packets.
Samara	75	10
Kazan...	75	10
Simbirsk.	75	10
Saratov..	75	10
Ufa....	75	10
Rostov-Don...	25	..
	400	50

In addition, the Rochester Community Chest donated food packets to a value of $5,000. A donation of $25,000 made by the Joint Distribution Committee was administered by the Medical Director, American Relief Administration in cooperation with the donor organization.

These packets served in many instances a three-fold purpose, relieving the acute food distress of the medical personnel, raising their morale and insured continuous Russian aid to the various special features of the American program. The Inoculation Campaign, the Clean-Up and Bathing Campaigns and work in connection with our dispensaries and the Roux Laboratory, were all made possible by this aid to physicians.

The clothing packets, which were issued at the close of our operation, were in tremendous demand. At this time acute food distress among medical personnel had been relieved but the extremely low salaries of physicians, nurses and feldshers, together with the high cost of all clothing, had made it impossible for them to renew their wardrobes. Practically all of them were wearing their patched up pre-war clothing.

-113-

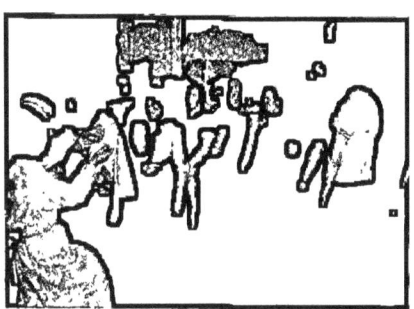 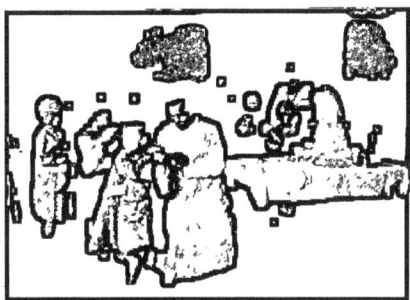

CHOLERA-TYPHOID INOCULATIONS

Left American sanitary unit inoculating repatriates passing through Petrograd, to prevent spread of disease into Central Europe *Right* Children being inoculated, which was compulsory for all children fed in American kitchens

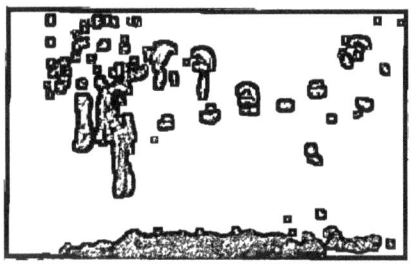 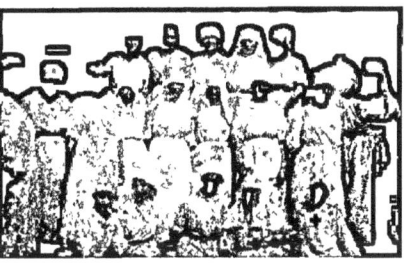

VOLGA REFUGEES WAITING THEIR TURN FOR INOCULATION

GROUP OF NURSES AT ROSTOV WHO INOCULATED 3,000 REFUGEES IN ONE DAY

THE INOCULATION CAMPAIGN

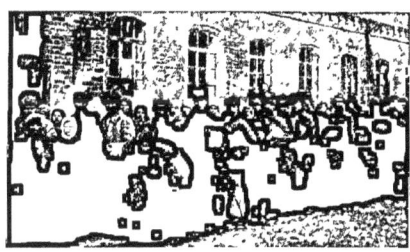 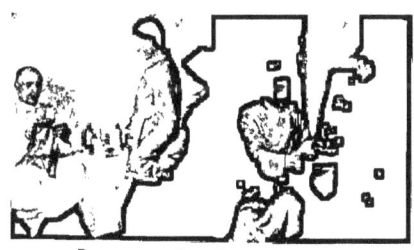

WAITING TURN AT A R A BATH HOUSE SAMARA

Where over 180,000 baths were given Note the birch branches with which bathers beat themselves

DISTRIBUTING SOAP BEFORE BATHING

THE BATHING CAMPAIGN AGAINST TYPHUS

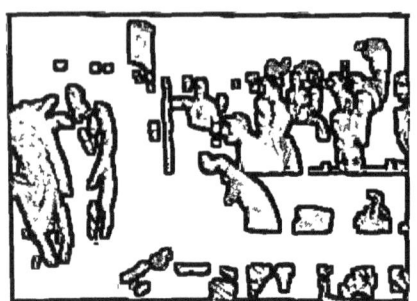

THE DRESSING ROOM

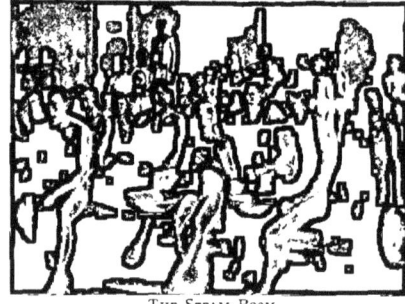

THE STEAM ROOM

INTERIOR OF A TYPICAL RUSSIAN BATH
The great mass of Russian people bathe in public bath houses not at home

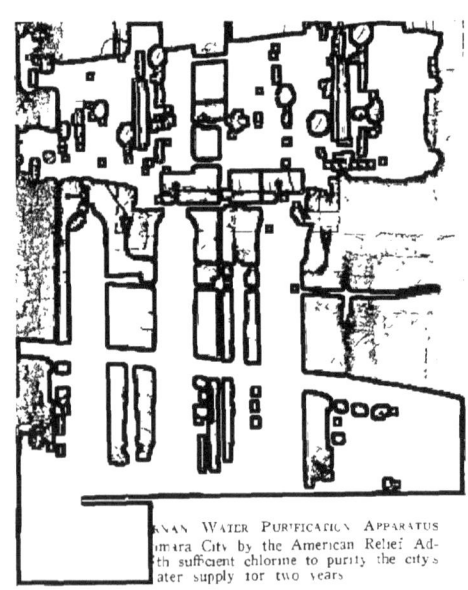

RUSSIAN WATER PURIFICATION APPARATUS
...mara City by the American Relief Ad-
...th sufficient chlorine to purify the city's
...ater supply for two years

CHAPTER XI.
SPECIAL MEASURES FOR PREVENTION OF DISEASE.
PURIFICATION OF WATER SUPPLY OF CITIES.

The purification plant of Orenburg city was completely overhauled, and sufficient quantities of alum and chloride of lime provided to purify its water supply during the summer of 1922. The water purification plant of Saratov city was likewise rehabilitated by labor receiving the American corn ration, and we made two issues of chloride of lime in sufficient quantities to purify the water used during the summers of 1922 and 1923. Large issues of this chemical were also made to the cities of Petrograd, Simbirsk, Nijni-Novgorod, Ekaterinoslav and Rostov-Don, which assured a pure water supply to these cities during the summers of 1922 and 1923. Over 1,000,000 pounds of chloride of lime were thus distributed. In addition, two complete sets of Wallace & Tiernan Chlorine Control Apparatus, purchased in America, were installed in the city of Samara, and a sufficient quantity of chlorine gas was provided to operate the apparatus for a period of approximately two years. This installation cost $16,000.

Large numbers of Lister Bags, with chemicals, were also distributed among the larger hospitals, children's homes and railroad stations, along routes of refugee movement.

Although usually equipped with water purification systems, most cities were unable to procure the necessary chemicals to operate them effectively and the water showed in consequence a high degree of contamination.

Resources did not permit the A.R.A. to do as much in this line as necessary, but what was done served materially to reduce disease in the cities mentioned.

SUPPLY OF DISINFECTORS.

A large disinfecting and bathing campaign, involving importation of the huge amounts of apparatus that would have been required, was entirely out of the question under the conditions pertaining in Russia, as shortage of water and fuel alone would have doomed this measure to failure. We felt, however, after consultations with the authorities in Moscow, that the importation of a number of large disinfectors for installation at important junction points was essential for refugees. We accordingly purchased six large French disinfecting camions, and installed them at refugee camps along the Western Russian frontier. Two of these were later withdrawn on urgent request of our district physicians and forwarded, one to Petrograd for the disinfecting of refugees' clothing, and the other to Samara for work at the Samara railroad station. All of this apparatus is now permanent equipment at refugee camps and infectious disease hospitals. The supply and rehabilitation of existing disinfecting units, plant for plant, was much cheaper than purchase of new equipment. Because of the limited funds available we accomplished much more service in this way than we could by capital expense of new equipment.

CLEAN-UP CAMPAIGNS.

During the spring of 1922, upon the arrival of the American corn, wide "Clean-Up Campaigns" were carried out in various districts. The workers in these campaigns were given the American corn ration. The most important work of these labor forces was removal of refuse from streets and the general cleaning of unsanitary conditions. Roads, bridges and public utilities were improved and repairs were made to hospitals and children's homes. This was especially the case in Ufa and Samara districts, where many hospitals and children's homes were entirely rehabilitated by our labor forces. Wood cutting detachments were also formed to secure fuel for hospitals and homes.

BATHING CAMPAIGN.

Many children receiving food in American kitchens and children's homes were filthy and infested with lice. Constant steps were taken to improve their hygiene. A bathing campaign was carried out in the Moscow district, in which free baths were provided for all of the children fed. In Odessa a large bath-house for children was opened where 2,600 were cleansed and their clothing disinfected on the first day While during the following three weeks 37,439 children and students from the University of Odessa were given at least one free bath.

A Bathing Campaign for children in the Samara district was carried out. Over 15,000 were bathed and their clothing disinfected. At a later period a free bath-house was established in Samara city where, during one hundred working days, the following groups received free baths.

Table 28

Laborers and office employees....	58,976
Poor and unemployed of Samara City..	102,222
Children from Children's Homes	11,817
Students from Samara University and other schools . . .	7,228
Children fed in A.R.A. Kitchens during April and May only..	762
	181,005

In addition, the clothing of 28,000 of the above was completely sterilized.

Throughout, a great improvement in the hygiene of the children was brought about, through inspection and insistence on reasonable standards of cleanliness. Soap was issued in most kitchens. In many, the children were made to wash their hands and faces before receiving their food.

THE INOCULATION CAMPAIGN.

Eight years of war, revolutions, counterrevolutions, famine, mass refugee movements, and increased poverty, had been prolific breeding seasons for widespread epidemics of insect borne diseases, such as typhus and relapsing fever, the water borne diseases as cholera, typhoid and paratyphoid fevers and various exanthemata, including smallpox.

Facilities for combatting disease and treating the sick, were deplorably limited when the American Relief Administration entered Russia, in September of 1921. From poverty many institutions were actually forced to close or curtail their operations at the very time when all facilities were most needed.

Temporary homes for refugees organized in famine areas in 1921, unheated and without any sanitary facilities, formed a distinct menace in the dissemination of disease. Shortage of fuel and water often made it impossible to hospitalize even infectious cases or delouse their effects and prevented operation of such disinfecting apparatus as existed. Bathing establishments were generally dismantled or out of commission due to lack of fuel. A considerable proportion of the people, especially in the provinces, was infested with lice.

Our early medical surveys revealed a poverty stricken people existing on scanty rations, living under the most unhygienic conditions, more or less riddled by constitutional disease; great epidemics of typhus, relapsing and typhoid fevers sweeping the country; cholera quiescent but threatening in the spring; twenty-four millions facing starvation; a great uncontrolled refugee mass carrying disease; and a medical famine existing throughout the whole of Russia; patients without clothing; beds with few blankets and no sheets; operating rooms with scanty dressings; pharmacies without essential medicines; kitchens with little food.

The American Relief Administration general medical program, which made possible improved sanitary conditions, and the prompt isolation and

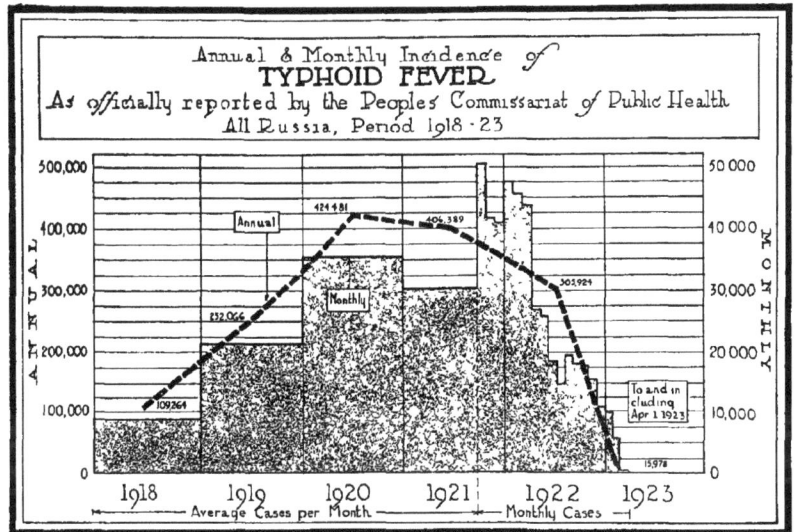

proper treatment of those suffering from infectious diseases, undoubtedly reduced the magnitude of epidemics, especially of typhus and relapsing fever. As inoculations and vaccinations afford the most effective method of preventing cholera, diseases of the typhoid group and smallpox in a country where sanitation can not be controlled we began early to formulate our plans for an extensive inoculation campaign so that as many as possible could be made immune to these diseases.

Vaccinations against smallpox and inoculations against cholera and typhoid fever are not by any means a new departure in Russia. The former is obligatory though not universally practiced due to shortage of vaccine and an inertia on the part of health authorities. The latter has been extensively carried out in the Red Army, and to a more limited extent among certain classes of workers, and travelers, but mass inoculation of the civilian population has never been attempted.

We will preface the report on the inoculation campaign with data of the registered cases of the various diseases. It must not be forgotten that

-118-

all Government figures are unreliable and that if reported cases are doubled or trebled they would, according to competent authorities, present a much more accurate picture of actual disease conditions.

Table 29
Typhoid Fever.

The number of cases officially reported are as follows:

1918, 109,264	1920, 424,481
1919, 252,066	1921, 406,389

1922, 305,924

The diagnosis of this disease is generally made upon the physical findings supported at times by the Widal test and Diazo reaction. In Russia, bacteriological examinations of the blood and the excreta are made only in some of the better class hospitals in larger cities and differentiation between typhoid and the paratyphoids is generally not made. Vaccines prepared in Russia do not include organisms of the paratyphoid group.

In every hospital one finds large numbers of cases of so-called "Status Typhosus" under which term are grouped undifferentiated typhus, typhoid, paratyphoid, relapsing fever and the various other diseases associated with fever. That there are so many of these undiagnosed cases is a sad commentary on the present state of medicine in Russia.

Smallpox.

This disease has always been more prevalent in Russia than in other countries of Europe. The number of cases even before the war averaged over 100,000 a year. According to Government statistics, no great increase in the morbidity rate incident took place to the world war, while the number of cases registered during the two years following the revolutions was very low. This was probably due to a more or less complete breakdown in the system for registering disease rather than to an actual decrease in the number of cases, for during 1919 when the administration of the statistical department had been improved, one hundred and sixty thousand cases were reported.

In April of 1920, the Commissioner of Public Health issued a decree making vaccination compulsory. This was followed by a considerable decrease in the morbidity rate, approximately ninety-eight thousand cases being registered in 1920 and eighty-five thousand in 1921.

In spite of the fact that vaccination is supposed to be compulsory, a large proportion of the population remains unprotected because of the impossibility of universally enforcing such a law under the conditions existing in Russia. In spite of the existence of numerous laboratories in larger cities, some of them very high class institutions, limited funds have kept them from operating to capacity. The amount of vaccines and sera, especially those requiring animal inoculation for their production (such as smallpox and diphtheria vaccine and meningococcic and dysentery serum) has been far below requirements. At the same time they have not been entirely satisfactory in quality. The A.R.A. had to augment the local supply by fairly large importations of these products. In carrying out our inoculation campaign, we had to vaccinate as many as possible against smallpox who have never been vaccinated before, as well as those who had not been revaccinated during recent years.

The following are the Government morbidity rates for smallpox for the last twelve years:

Table 30

1910,	165,000;	1913,	72,000;	1916,	105,000;	1919,	158,747;
1911,	119,000;	1914,	94,162;	1917,	65,000;	1920,	96,475;
1912,	81,000;	1915,	121,000;	1918,	55,956;	1921,	85,716;
			1922,	58,473.			

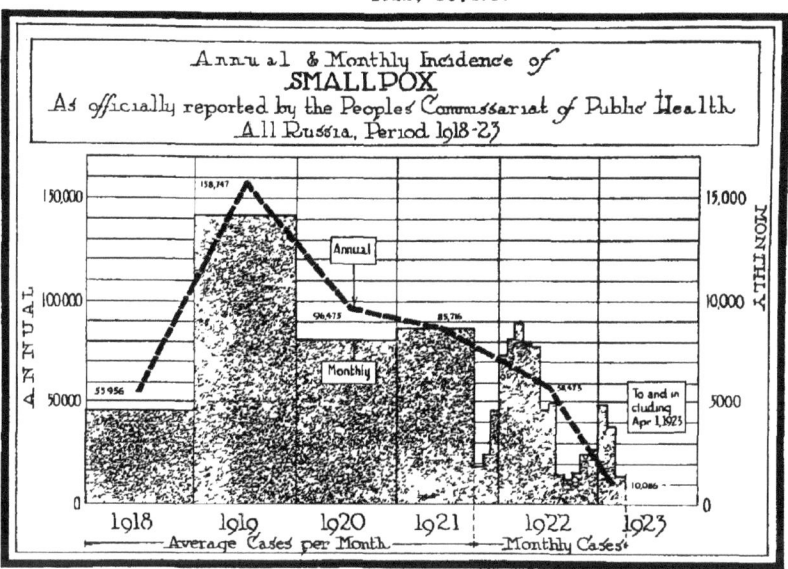

Annual & Monthly Incidence of
SMALLPOX
As officially reported by the Peoples' Commissariat of Public Health
All Russia, Period 1918-23

Cholera.

This disease, which has almost been eliminated from other parts of Europe, has appeared during the summer of each year of the present century with the exception of 1903 and 1906. The number of cases has, however, varied markedly from a minimum of nine in 1912 to a maximum of over six hundred thousand in 1892. A study of the cholera statistics for the last hundred years reveals the fact that the average number of cases shows little decrease during the last century. The persistence of the preventable diseases, such as cholera and smallpox in Russia furnishes an index of the poor sanitary conditions and of the indifference and ignorance of the people.

Statistics for cholera are very much more accurate than are those for typhoid fever because the disease is much more spectacular and receives greater attention because of the high mortality. The diagnosis is based on bacteriological findings in a large percentage of cases.

Cholera is endemic in Southeastern Russia where the disease remains latent during the winter months. Epidemics of greater magnitude, which begin usually in early spring, involve all sections of southern and central Russia and even areas in the north. The disease has a tendency to appear suddenly, in a particular locality, reach a maximum very rapidly and then die out and reappear in another section. It has been pointed out that the epidemic rarely strikes the same area in succeeding years and that territories which have experienced a maximum of cases during one epidemic year would appear to be relatively immune for a considerable period thereafter

Though cholera is a constant menace, the actual number of cases occurring from year to year in Russia is not nearly so great as one might expect in a country where all conditions are so favorable for its development and spread. Previous to the A.R.A. issue of chloride of lime last summer, cholera vibrios were demonstrated in the water supply of Petrograd city. The great majority of people secure their water from shallow wells, frequently sunk in polluted areas and without any attempt being made to protect the surrounding terrain. Food is handled in a filthy manner with every opportunity for contamination, while personal hygiene does not receive much attention from the average peasant. In spite of this, the average number of cases has remained low as compared with other intestinal diseases. The incidence was not materially increased during the recent years of war, and though the epidemics of the last two years have claimed many victims, they are not to be compared from the point of view of numbers with those of typhoid, typhus and relapsing fever.

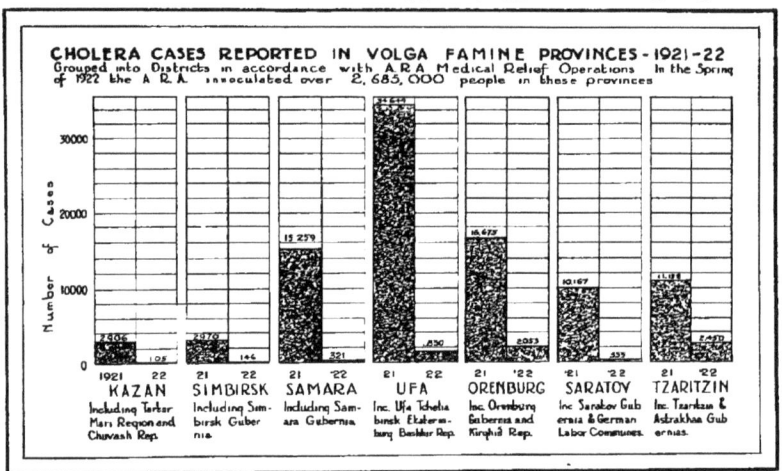

There is therefore either a great decrease of resistance on the part of the Russian people to the cholera vibrio or a markedly attenuated organism. Minorov and Belayevtsev demonstrated by the Pfeiffer reaction, that approximately two-thirds of the population of Krasnodar possess a certain degree of immunity to the cholera vibrio. In connection with this immunity, carriers may be important. At Professor Kershuni's laboratory at Kharkov it has been demonstrated that the blood serum of carriers possesses antibodies similar to those acquired through an attack of the disease. "Carriers" are either mild, ambulatory cases or individuals who have recovered from an attack of the disease.

The epidemics at their onset are undoubtedly water-borne in many places as indicated by positive bacteriological examinations of the water supply. Once an epidemic has begun, however, the great majority of cases are probably transmitted by contact. Large numbers of carriers are always discov-

ered where the disease prevails. These carriers, and especially latent foci
in southeast Russia are responsible for the reinfection of the country from
year to year. Two main foci exist: (1) Tashkent via railroad through Orenburg, (2) Persia through Afghanistan via Volga region. The refugee movement
has played an important role in the spread of the infection throughout Russia.

The following figures indicate the average prevalence of this
disease: 1914, 10,555; 1915, 55,000; 1916, 3,080; 1917, 41,352; 1918, 41,128;
1919, 7,719; 1920, 32,000; 1921, 176,885. The average mortality has run between fifty and sixty per cent. Years of famine are associated with a great increase in the disease; in 1892, 620,000 cases were reported; in 1910 there
were over 230,000 cases. The cholera epidemic of 1921 when 176,885 cases were
reported, was a deadly visitation involving all parts of Russia but with a
preponderance of cases in the Volga Basin, approximately 93,904 occurring
there. We realized that a repetition of the scourge was inevitable during

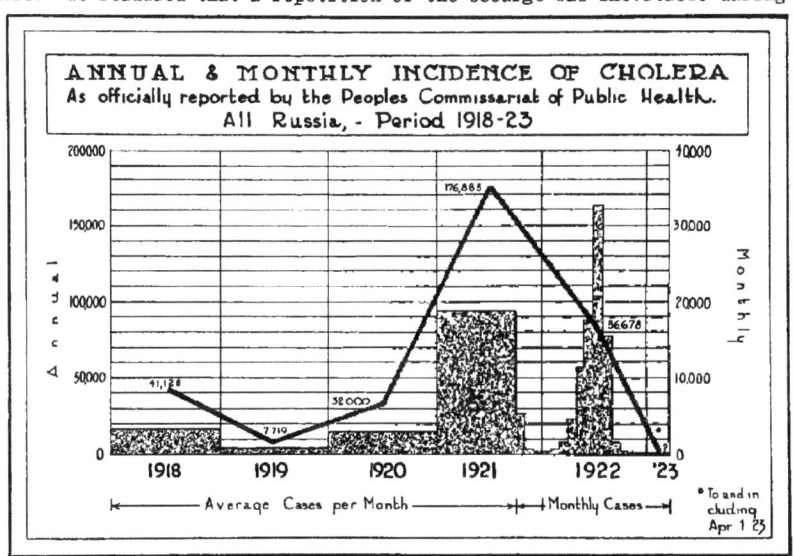

ANNUAL & MONTHLY INCIDENCE OF CHOLERA
As officially reported by the Peoples Commissariat of Public Health.
All Russia, - Period 1918-23

the summer of 1922, and feared that its magnitude might even be greater than
during the previous year, especially along the Volga, where famine had lowered
the resistance of the inhabitants.

The Inoculation Campaign.

To combat this foreseen cholera epidemic and at the same time to protect the population against other water-borne diseases the A.R.A. decided on
a mass inoculation campaign in all our districts, which included, at that
time, Moscow, Petrograd, Kazan, Simbirsk, Samara, Saratov, Tzaritzin, Ufa
and Orenburg, covering in addition to Moscow and Petrograd, the entire "famine
area" and the territory to the east as far as the border of Siberia. We aimed
to inoculate all children whom we were feeding, as many as possible of the
adults who were receiving our corn rations, and in addition, all others who
desired this protective inoculation.

As the expense incident to the purchase of vaccines, syringes and other materials for a campaign of this kind was considerable, we did not undertake it before making a thorough investigation as to its practicability and probability of success. Numerous personnel would be required. The difficulties and labor involved in distributing materials and carrying out inoculations among some millions of persons scattered over a wide area would be great. We apprehended, in addition, considerable opposition to the measure because those whom we proposed to inoculate were, as a rule, ignorant, superstitious, and fearful of surgery. But the general population became quite worried at the imminence of cholera and were reported as anxious to protect themselves against the disease. American feeding supervisors assured us that their control over both adults and children who were receiving the American Relief Administration ration would assure the success of the campaign.

Because only a limited amount of divaccine (i. e. typhoid--cholera vaccine) was being prepared at a few of the Government laboratories, it would be necessary for us to provide the bulk of vaccines needed as well as to furnish all other materials needed for the work. We had already made tentative arrangements with the Pasteur Institute Paris, through the London Office of the American Relief Administration, to manufacture large quantities of tetra-vaccine containing the following organisms per cubic centimeter:

Cholera............	4,000,000,000
Typhoid.......	1,800,000,000
Para-Typhoid A....	1,250,000,000
Para-Typhoid B.................	1,250,000,000

A course of this vaccine for an adult consists of two doses given at seven to ten days intervals, the first dose for an adult being one cubic centimeter and second dose double this amount

Upon our decision to inaugurate the campaign, we immediately placed an order with the Institute for 2,000,000 cubic centimeters of this vaccine. We ordered 1,000,000 doses of small-pox vaccine at the same time. Large numbers of syringes were also purchased. As needs developed and as the success of the operation was assured, we placed additional orders. In all, 7,000,000 cubic centimeters of Tetra-Vaccine, 1,000,000 doses of Mono-Vaccine and 3,500,000 doses of Small-Pox vaccine were purchased.

The Pasteur Institute enjoys the highest reputation among medical men in Russia and as we wished to obviate all possible criticism of the vaccines which we used and as we were promised expeditious deliveries at a price very much lower than that quoted by firms in America, we used only their product throughout the campaign. Vaccines were all shipped from Paris to Moscow and again from Moscow to our various district headquarters by special couriers. This insured prompt and rapid deliveries. Cholera was already appearing and early immunization against the disease was imperative. This arrangement proved very satisfactory, and enabled us to keep district personnel supplied with vaccines almost uninterruptedly from April 20th, when the first shipments arrived, up to the time the campaign was completed.

For administrative purposes we divided all of the area in which the A.R.A. was carrying out relief work, with a population of roughly eighty millions, into districts. These districts frequently included several gubernias or republics and were again divided into sub-districts or regions with local personnel and warehouses. In villages we had committees made up of the more prominent citizens generally including a physician. As all district and sub-district as well as village personnel were under our immediate control, this organization provided a ready and effective means for securing information, and for distributing, checking, and accounting for food and medical supplies. It also made possible the prompt inoculation and vaccination of great numbers of individuals scattered over a very wide area.

We relied upon the resourcefulness and ingenuity of our physicians to develop the most effective methods for carrying out the details of the campaign. We made inoculations compulsory for all children who were being fed as well as for all adults receiving our corn ration only exempting the sick and those in very poor physical condition. This compulsory feature of our plan probably furnished the greatest factor in its success as it eliminated delay and made possible the protection of that element of the population we were most anxious to render immune.

Inoculations in Country Districts.

District physicians perfected their plans for carrying out the work locally either with or independently of the Government, so that upon the arrival of vaccines they promptly began work.

We equipped all Medical Institutions with inoculation material, and established special inoculation dispensaries as well, hoping thereby to reach a greater number of the general population. To reach the children every district organized inoculation "teams."

In the Saratov District, Dr. Toole used large numbers of medical students from the fourth and fifth year classes of the Saratov University. Upon the arrival of a consignment of vaccine, he sent out a squad of these students, under control of an inspector-physician, to a vaccination area corresponding to a child-feeding area. Each squad took with it the vaccine, necessary syringes, iodine, alcohol, cotton and a medical chest. The Sub-District was divided among the various students who visited in turn all towns and villages where the American Relief Administration kitchens were located. With the assistance of local physicians, feldshers and nurses, they examined the children and inoculated all whose physical condition would permit. As each student's area was very large, it required from seven to ten days to cover all towns, so that the final inoculations were due upon the completion of the preliminary circuit, and it required approximately three weeks to complete the work in a given area. Large numbers of students were available, so that the nine vaccination areas of our Saratov District were covered in short order. In all over 330,000 persons were thus vaccinated and inoculated.

In the Samara District, Dr. Foucar organized one hundred and sixty vaccinating companies, each composed of one doctor and a feldsher. He appointed inspectors for each region who controlled the work and instructed the personnel of companies in the proper use of the materials supplied. This district embraced nine "Regions" with 1792 kitchens feeding over 400,000 children. His returns showed over 400,000 inoculated.

Local Government Officials as a rule cooperated satisfactorily. In the vast Ufa District the whole-hearted support from officials alone made possible the inoculation of 931,000. This district made inoculations compulsory for the following classes:

    1. All government employees.

    2. All children fed at American kitchens.

    3. Children and adults in government institutions.

    4. Persons receiving the corn ration from the American Relief Administration.

    5. All persons travelling either by road or railroad were required

to have a certificate of inoculation.

Similarly in Kazan, where over 600,000 persons received primary inoculations, and where 420,000 persons were vaccinated, Dr. Dear operated in close harmony with the President of the Tartar Republic and local Government Officials.

The work in Moscow and Petrograd was carried out rapidly. Though we supplied vaccine to institutions for protecting the general population and volunteers, our teams inoculated only the children receiving American Relief Administration food and certain refugee elements, making a total in the two cities of approximately 93,000.

During the spring of 1922 we established the medical relief districts of Kiev, Kharkov, Odessa and Alexandrovsk, covering the entire Ukraine, the district of Minsk for White Russia, Theodosia for the Crimea, and Rostov for Southeastern Russia extending southward to the Caucasus. Liberal supplies of vaccines and materials required for making inoculations were issued all these districts and the campaign was carried out as vigorously as possible by our physicians in charge. However, as feeding had not yet begun on a large scale, and as district organizations were not perfected until late spring or early summer, the epidemic of cholera had developed widely before preventative work could be initiated. Large numbers were nevertheless inoculated and vaccinated as indicated in the summary given below.

The program received considerable publicity from local newspapers. Numerous articles explained the benefits derived from vaccination and inoculation. They helped to create a favorable attitude on the part of the peasants. We quote one such from the "Sickle and Hammer," Saratov.

THE WORK OF THE AMERICAN RELIEF ADMINISTRATION IN THE DISTRICT

Once more a squad of the American Relief Administration has come to our Serdobak to vaccinate the population, this time against smallpox, cholera and typhoid. To make the work of the American Relief Administration squad successful, unanimous propaganda on the part of the cultured population of the village is absolutely necessary. Units of R K P (Bolsheveks), Volispolcoms, Soviets of the villages, and local intelligentsia must all do this work.

It is not necessary to repeat the facts proving that vaccination, while harmless for the body, make it unsusceptible to certain diseases. For instance, in the city of Serdobak the squad of the American Relief Administration did 4,096 smallpox vaccinations and 3,112 initial inoculations against abdominal typhus and 2,490 second inoculations. Not one of the citizens suffered from inoculation, and they all feel very well and comfortable, being afraid neither of cholera nor smallpox.

Of course we understand perfectly well that the time of cholera-mutinies on the part of ignorant peasants has passed, that our village has made great progress during the revolutionary period. Peasants who took part in the war saw life in Germany and Austria and learned to love culture. Therefore, we are sure that the work of the American Relief Administration will be successful, but all kinds of co-operation must be rendered in the field to the squad.

The squad of the American Relief Administration under Dr Kopernaumov, sent from Saratov by Dr Toole, will visit at first the large villages of our ouyezd. They propose to do 20,000 vaccinations against smallpox and typhoid.

Smallpox vaccinations to school age children are compulsory as they were in Serdobak.

The squad has some soap which will be distributed to the poorest population to improve the anti-sanitary conditions of their life.

Vaccinations are the achievement of high culture.

Peasants of the ouyezd, avail yourselves of the relief of the American Relief Administration.

-125-

An interesting feature, in connection with the campaign, is the fact that practically no expense was incurred, either on the part of the Soviet Government or the American Relief Administration, for payment of medical personnel who made inoculations. We had received a gift of $35,000 from Mr William Bingham, 2d, of Boston for food packets for medical personnel We distributed many of these packets to poverty-stricken physicians and feldshers, who, in lieu of other payment, assisted us in carrying out inoculations The packets, therefore, served a double purpose and were a tremendously important factor in the success of the campaign

SUMMARY OF INOCULATIONS AND VACCINATIONS.

The figures quoted below, represent, by districts, the inoculations and vaccinations carried out during the spring, autumn and early fall of 1922 under the direction of the Medical Division of the American Relief Administration.

Table 31

District.	Small-pox Vaccinations Completed.	Tetra Inoculations, 1st Dose.	Completed Tetra Inoculations, 2nd Dose.
Kazan	230,065	604,482	383,074
Simbirsk	84,161	259,195	259,195
Samara	42,966	400,488	399,522
Orenburg	36,837	80,000	80,000
Ufa	41,589	931,928	931,928
Saratov	331,977	331,668	315,709
Tzaritzin.	78,000	78,000	78,000
Total Inoculations for the famine area, 5,133,149.			
Kharkov	....	160,500	160,500
Odessa	94,089	115,664	87,899
Kiev	134,000	112,000	81,000
Ekaterinoslav	115,000	149,500	149,500
Minsk	132,000	51,000	51,000
Rostov	195,000	195,000	160,000
Simferopol	20,615	44,000	44,000
Moscow.	26,639	46,480	44,697
Petrograd	27,198	42,285	45,000
Totals, all Russia	1,590,136	3,602,190	3,271,024

These figures do not include inoculations and vaccinations against typhoid fever and small-pox carried out with our supplies previous to the initiation of the campaign, or large numbers of vaccinations performed during the winter with our vaccine.

We reinaugurated the campaign during the spring of 1923 among children fed by the American Relief Administration not previously protected.

Also, we continued to issue materials for inoculations wherever indicated and restocked several districts which were not in position to prepare vaccine needed locally. Considerable quantities of laboratory supplies were also issued and we trust that laboratories of Russia will be in a position in future to prepare necessary vaccines for carrying out preventive inoculation.

Results.--A study of the comparative incidence of cholera for all of Russia and for the districts in which the American Relief Administration is operating is suggestive.

Table 32

Incidence of Cholera All Russia 1921 and 1922.

Total number cases reported 1921..... 176,885
Total number cases reported 1922.......... 86,675

Total number of cases of cholera reported in famine provinces Volga region 1921 and 1922* grouped into districts in accordance with Medical Relief Operations.

Table 33

District	Territory.	1921.	1922.
Kazan... .	Tartar, Marisk and Tchouvash Republics..	2,906	105
Simbirsk. .	Simbirsk, Penza, Nijni-Novgorod..	2,970	146
Samara .	Samara..	15,259	321
Ufa........	Ufa, Cheliabinsk, Ekaterinburg, Bashkir Republic	34,649	1,830
Orenburg	Orenburg, Kirghiz Republic...	16,675	2,053
Saratov....	Saratov, German Labor Commune	10,167	355
Tzaritzin..	Tzaritzin, Astrakhan..	11,158	2,450
	Total...........	93,784	7,260

It will be noted from the above that the number of cases of cholera which occurred during 1922 was approximately one-half the reported incidence of the previous year, while in the Volga area, where we began our inoculation campaign early and where we carried it out most intensively, the incidence fell from 93,784 to 7,260. In the Ukraine, where our campaign began at a much later date and where due to the recent development of our organization, it could not be carried out as effectively or promptly, cholera cases reached 41,896 as compared with 10,341 during the previous year.

In spite of the fact that probably many were rendered immune to cholera in the Volga area during the summer of 1921, when 93,784 cases of cholera occurred, we were extremely apprehensive lest an epidemic of even greater proportions should visit this region during the summer of 1922. The incidence of cholera is always liable to be very high during famine years, and the famine in Russia was centered in this area.

As very many factors come into play in connection with the epidemiology of disease, we are loath to draw any radical conclusions from the above figures. We believed the improvement in the water supply, and in general sanitary conditions, the issue to all hospitals and homes of drugs, medicines and necessary supplies to allow them to function and permit early isolation and treatment of the sick, as well as the inoculation campaign mentioned above, were most important factors in preventing a huge epidemic in the area in question. In this connection it should be remembered that the inoculations were carried out in the main among the poorer and more ignorant classes and that this element of the population is most prone to contract and disseminate infectious diseases.

A few special instances of the limitation of cholera by inoculation deserve mention. In the city of Samara during June, after the beginning of our Inoculation Campaign, an average of only two new cases per week were reported, while previous to that time the incidence had been higher and the abnormally early appearance of the disease threatened an epidemic. In Saratov

*The American Relief Administration Inoculation Campaign was conducted during the spring and summer, 1922.

city the beginning of an epidemic of cholera induced Dr. Toole to carry out a very rapid and intensive inoculation campaign. The disease entirely disappeared on completion of the same.

Our data is as yet very incomplete as to the number of individuals developing cholera after inoculations. The report of Dr. Dear for the city of Kazan, however, shows that among 57,564 vaccinated persons only twenty-three developed cholera, whereas among 88,692 unvaccinated individuals there were 253 cases of the disease, and that the death rate among vaccinated reached approximately forty per cent. as compared with fifty-two per cent. for the unvaccinated. In Samara District no cases of cholera were reported from among those vaccinated; the cases registered for 1922 occurred mainly among transients arriving from other parts.

As to the results of this campaign in controlling typhoid fever, though data is incomplete, we received reports from Samara, however, that the incidence of this disease in that region where over 400,000 persons were inoculated was almost nil. The rate in all our Volga districts was very much lower at the termination of our activities than during previous years.

It is believed that the American Administration inoculation campaign which rendered almost four million persons relatively immune to cholera, and absolutely immune to typhoid and para-typhoid, and which protected, as well, very large numbers against small-pox, materially reduced the magnitude of the cholera epidemic in the summer of 1922. Undoubtedly, as well, the successful carrying out of the measure in spite of many difficulties and some opposition, has had a marked effect upon the medical profession and has stimulated them to new efforts. Its importance from a general educational point of view should not be forgotten.

The campaign was instituted as an emergency measure and carried out by personnel who were not trained in epidemiological work, with great rapidity and over a vast territory. Studies relative to serological results of inoculations were not possible and accurate statistics as to comparative morbidity and mortality rates among the inoculated and non-inoculated population will never be available. This is regretted, but neither the purpose nor the possibilities of this campaign were to gather scientific data. It was to limit the incidence of small-pox and water-borne diseases among a famine-stricken people.

Although the coming of the 1922 harvest brought an end to the necessity of feeding millions of famine sufferers by importation of American supplies, the famine left in its train undernourishment, weakness, and susceptibility to disease and epidemics which made necessary the carrying on of the American medical program through the year of famine aftermath.

Even in spite of the great amount of American medical supplies imported and distributed, and in spite of all these efforts of medical relief, disinfection, and sanitation, the Russian people still had much lost ground to gain in rehabilitation of medical practice. But the worst period had been covered. It was deemed that America had done her share and could withdraw, leaving the Russian Government to carry on by its own efforts.

Its work done, the last contingent of American physicians left Moscow for home early in July 1923.